Cutting-Edge Medicine

What Psychiatrists Need to Know

Review of Psychiatry Series
John M. Oldham, M.D., M.S.
Michelle B. Riba, M.D., M.S.
Series Editors

Cutting-Edge Medicine

What Psychiatrists Need to Know

EDITED BY

Nada L. Stotland, M.D., M.P.H.

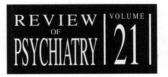

REVIEW OF PSYCHIATRY | VOLUME 21

No. 1

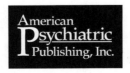

American Psychiatric Publishing, Inc.

Washington, DC
London, England

Note: The authors have worked to ensure that all information in this book concerning drug dosages, schedules, and routes of administration is accurate as of the time of publication and consistent with standards set by the U.S. Food and Drug Administration and the general medical community. As medical research and practice advance, however, therapeutic standards may change. For this reason and because human and mechanical errors sometimes occur, we recommend that readers follow the advice of a physician who is directly involved in their care or the care of a member of their family. A product's current package insert should be consulted for full prescribing and safety information.

Books published by American Psychiatric Publishing, Inc., represent the views and opinions of the individual authors and do not necessarily represent the policies and opinions of APPI or the American Psychiatric Association.

Copyright © 2002 American Psychiatric Publishing, Inc.

07   06   05   04   03   7   6   5   4   3   2

ALL RIGHTS RESERVED

Manufactured in the United States of America on acid-free paper

American Psychiatric Publishing, Inc.
1000 Wilson Boulevard, Suite 1825
Arlington, VA 22209
www.appi.org

The correct citation for this book is

Stotland NL (editor): *Cutting-Edge Medicine: What Psychiatrists Need to Know* (Review of Psychiatry Series, Volume 21, Number 1; Oldham JM and Riba MB, series editors). Washington, DC, American Psychiatric Publishing, 2002

Library of Congress Cataloging-in-Publication Data

Cutting-edge medicine : what psychiatrists need to know / edited by Nada L. Stotland.
     p. ; cm. — (Review of psychiatry; v. 21, 1)
   Includes bibliographical referencesand index.
   ISBN 1-58562-072-6 (alk. paper)
    1. Mental illness. 2. Comorbidity. 3. Transplantation of organs, tissues,
  etc.—Psychological aspects. 4. Psychiatry. I. Stotland, Nada Logan. II. Review of
psychiatry series ; v. 21, 1.
     [DNLM: 1. Mental Disorders—complications. 2. Cardiovascular
Diseases—complications. 3. Comorbidity. 4. Digestive System Diseases—
complications.
   5. Menstruation Disturbances—complications. 6. Organ Transplantation—psychology.
WM 140 C9912 2002]
   RC480.5 .C884 2002
   616 89—dc21

                                                               2001058387

British Library Cataloguing in Publication Data
A CIP record is available from the British Library.

Contents

Chapter 3
Psychiatric Overview of Solid
Organ Transplantation

Catherine C. Crone, M.D.
Geoffrey Gabriel, M.D.

Chapter 4
Psychiatric Disorders and the Menstrual Cycle

Laura J. Miller, M.D.

Index

Contributors

Catherine C. Crone, M.D.
Staff Psychiatrist, Inova Transplant Center, Falls Church, Virginia; Associate Clinical Professor of Psychiatry, Georgetown University Medical Center, Washington, D.C.

Steven A. Epstein, M.D.
Associate Professor and Interim Chair, Department of Psychiatry, Georgetown University Hospital, Washington, D.C.

Geoffrey Gabriel, M.D.
Chief, Inpatient Psychiatry, 121st General Army Hospital, Seoul, Korea

Ahmed Sherif Meguid, M.B., Ch.B.
Clinical Lecturer, Department of Psychiatry, University of Saskatchewan, Saskatoon, Saskatchewan, Canada

Laura J. Miller, M.D.
Associate Professor and Chief, Women's Services Division, Department of Psychiatry, University of Illinois at Chicago, Chicago, Illinois

John M. Oldham, M.D., M.S.
Dollard Professor and Acting Chairman, Department of Psychiatry, Columbia University College of Physicians and Surgeons, New York, New York

John Querques, M.D.
Attending Psychiatrist, Erich Lindemann Mental Health Center; Clinical Assistant in Psychiatry, Massachusetts General Hospital; Instructor in Psychiatry, Harvard Medical School, Boston, Massachusetts

Michelle B. Riba, M.D., M.S.
Associate Chair for Education and Academic Affairs, Department of Psychiatry, University of Michigan Medical School, Ann Arbor, Michigan

Theodore A. Stern, M.D.
Psychiatrist and Chief, The Avery D. Weisman, M.D., Psychiatry Consultation Service, Massachusetts General Hospital; Associate Professor of Psychiatry, Harvard Medical School, Boston, Massachusetts

Nada L. Stotland, M.D., M.P.H.
Professor, Departments of Psychiatry and Obstetrics/Gynecology, Rush Medical College, Chicago, Illinois

Thomas N. Wise, M.D.
Medical Director, Behavioral Health Services, and Chairman, Department of Psychiatry, Inova Fairfax Hospital, Falls Church, Virginia; Professor and Vice Chair, Department of Psychiatry, Georgetown University School of Medicine, Washington, D.C.

Introduction to the Review of Psychiatry Series

John M. Oldham, M.D., M.S., and
Michelle B. Riba, M.D., M.S., Series Editors

2002 REVIEW OF PSYCHIATRY SERIES TITLES

- *Cutting-Edge Medicine: What Psychiatrists Need to Know*
  EDITED BY NADA L. STOTLAND, M.D., M.P.H.
- *The Many Faces of Depression in Children and Adolescents*
  EDITED BY DAVID SHAFFER, F.R.C.P.(LOND), F.R.C.PSYCH.(LOND),
  AND BRUCE D. WASLICK, M.D.
- *Emergency Psychiatry*
  EDITED BY MICHAEL H. ALLEN, M.D.
- *Mental Health Issues in Lesbian, Gay, Bisexual, and Transgender Communities*
  EDITED BY BILLY E. JONES, M.D., M.S., AND MARJORIE J. HILL, PH.D.

There is a growing literature describing the stress–vulnerability model of illness, a model applicable to many, if not most, psychiatric disorders and to physical illness as well. Vulnerability comes in a number of forms. Genetic predisposition to specific conditions may arise as a result of spontaneous mutations, or it may be transmitted intergenerationally in family pedigrees. Secondary types of vulnerability may involve susceptibility to disease caused by the weakened resistance that accompanies malnutrition, immunocompromised states, and other conditions. In most of these models of illness, vulnerability consists of a necessary but not sufficient precondition; if specific stresses are avoided, or if they are encountered but offset by adequate protective factors, the disease does not manifest itself and the vulnerability may never be recognized. Conversely, there is increasing recognition of the role of stress as a precipitant of frank illness in vulnerable individuals and of the complex and subtle interactions among the environment, emotions, and neurodevelopmental, metabolic, and physiological processes.

In this country, the years 2001 and 2002 contained stress of unprecedented proportions, with the terrorist attacks on September 11 and the events that followed that terrible day. Although the contents of Volume 21 of the Review of Psychiatry were well established by that date and much of the text had already been written, we could not introduce this volume without thinking about the relevance of this unanticipated, widespread stress to the topics already planned.

Certainly, major depression is one of the prime candidates among the disorders in vulnerable populations that can be precipitated by stress. The information presented in *The Many Faces of Depression in Children and Adolescents,* edited by David Shaffer and Bruce D. Waslick, is, then, timely indeed. Already identified as a growing problem in youth—all too often accompanied by suicidal behavior—depression in children and adolescents is especially important to identify as early as possible. School-based screening services need to be widespread in order to facilitate both prevention of the disorder in those at risk and referral for effective treatment for those already experiencing symptomatic depression. Both psychotherapy and pharmacotherapy are well established as effective treatments for this condition, making recognition of its presence even more important. In New York alone, thousands of children lost at least one parent in the World Trade Center disaster, a catastrophic event precipitating not just grief but also major depression in the children and adolescents at risk.

We now know that stress, and depression itself, affect not just the brain but the body as well. New information about this brain–body axis is provided in *Cutting-Edge Medicine: What Psychiatrists Need to Know,* edited by Nada L. Stotland. Depression as an independent risk factor for cardiac death is one of the new findings reviewed in the chapter on the mind and the heart, as we understand more about the interactions among emotions, behavior, and cardiovascular functioning. Similarly, stress and mood are primary players in the homeostasis, or lack of it, of other body systems, such as the menstrual cycle and gastrointestinal functioning, also reviewed in this book. Finally, the massive increase in organ transplantation, in which medical advances have made it possible to neutralize the body's own immune responses against foreign tissue, represents a new frontier in which emotional stability is critical in donor and recipient.

Increasingly, medicine's front door is the hospital emergency service. Not just a place where triage occurs, though that remains an important and challenging function, the psychiatric emergency service needs to have expert clinicians who can perform careful assessments and initiate treatment. The latest thinking by psychiatrists experienced in emergency work is presented in *Emergency Psychiatry*, edited by Michael H. Allen. Certainly, psychiatric emergency services serve as one of the most critical components of the response network that needs to be in place to deal with a disaster such as the September 2001 attack and the bioterrorism events that followed.

Perhaps less obviously linked to those September events, *Mental Health Issues in Lesbian, Gay, Bisexual, and Transgender Communities*, edited by Billy E. Jones and Marjorie J. Hill, which reviews current thinking about gay, lesbian, bisexual, and transgender issues, reflects our changing world in other ways. A continuing process is necessary as we rethink our assumptions and challenge and question any prejudice or bias that may have infiltrated our thinking or may have been embedded in our traditional concepts. In this book, traditional notions are contrasted with newer thinking about gender role and sexual orientation, considering these issues from youth to old age, as we continue to try to differentiate the wide range of human diversity from what we classify as illness.

We believe that the topics covered in Volume 21 are timely and represent a selection of important updates for the practicing clinician. Next year, this tradition will continue, with books on trauma and disaster response and management, edited by Robert J. Ursano and Ann E. Norwood; on molecular neurobiology for the clinician, edited by Dennis S. Charney; on geriatric psychiatry, edited by Alan M. Mellow; and on standardized assessment for the clinician, edited by Michael B. First.

Preface

Nada L. Stotland, M.D., M.P.H.

Psychosomatic medicine has been a preoccupation of physicians and nonphysicians since ancient times. Hippocrates blamed symptoms we now see as psychiatric on a wandering uterus. During the lifetimes of many mid-career mental health professionals, we have seen a major evolution of theory and practice at the interface of physical symptoms, general medical diseases, and psychiatry. Fifty years ago, psychiatrists had identified the personality profiles and unconscious conflicts that caused ulcer disease, asthma, and rheumatoid arthritis. The connections seemed to be confirmed not only in clinical experience but also by personality tests and other research procedures. It did not occur to most of us until years later that the psychological attributes we were observing in these patients might be secondary to their years of suffering with serious, potentially fatal diseases.

During the late sixties and the seventies of the last century, in many major medical centers, consultation-liaison psychiatrists were assigned to each medical subspecialty. In some cases, psychiatrists became persona non grata on medical floors, blamed for assigning a psychiatric diagnosis to every patient, exacerbating patients' symptoms by stirring up feelings in vulnerable areas, writing lengthy reports incomprehensible to the referring staff, and recommending psychoanalytic psychotherapy for whatever ailed the patient. One of the supervising consultation-liaison psychiatrists during my training chastised the residents for wearing white coats on the medical/surgical floors, reminding us that, in order to become good psychiatrists after our years of medical school and our internships, we would now have to unlearn the medical model.

That sounds ridiculous now, but historical observations shouldn't make us smug. Decades from now, our successors will find our theories and practices equally laughable. The lesson is that medicine is a living and evolving profession. In recent years, psychiatrists have reclaimed our medical identity—the unique training that enables us to recognize, grasp, study, and utilize the mind-body connections that are currently the focus of some of the most exciting discoveries in the history of humankind. We are back in the game. The American Psychiatric Association has acted favorably on a proposal that psychosomatic medicine be considered an official subspecialty of psychiatry.

Our psychosomatic experts serve several crucial functions. As they help our non-psychiatric colleagues with the psychiatric aspects of their research and clinical care, they can keep the mental health professions informed about cutting-edge issues in other branches of medicine. This volume is part of that effort. Psychiatrists who work with gynecologists, gastroenterologists, cardiologists, and organ transplant teams have contributed chapters bringing together and synthesizing the latest in diagnosis, etiology, pathophysiology, and treatment. Their chapters are rigorously researched, intellectually stimulating, and clinically useful. I commend them to the reader.

Chapter 1

Mind and Heart

The Interplay Between Psychiatric and Cardiac Illness

John Querques, M.D.
Theodore A. Stern, M.D.

The heart—the seat of love and passion, and perhaps even the soul—is endowed with special psychological significance by the layperson. Common expressions attest to this lofty position occupied by the heart: one who is outwardly emotional is said to wear his or her heart on his or her sleeve, and the cause of death of someone whose longtime companion has recently died is attributed to a broken heart. Examples from poetry and folklore of the inextricable link between human moods and the heart are ample (Glassman and Shapiro 1998). The medical and psychiatric literature has lagged behind the common vernacular and poets' musings, but research evidence linking the mind (i.e., the brain) and the heart is burgeoning.

Cardiovascular disease is the leading cause of death in the United States and a significant source of morbidity. According to the National Health and Nutrition Examination Survey III (Centers for Disease Control and Prevention and American Heart Association 1996), nearly 61 million Americans—nearly one in five—have some form of cardiovascular disease. Coronary artery disease (CAD) accounts for almost 12.5 million of these cases. In addition, psychiatric disorders are similarly prevalent among the American populace, with depression afflicting approximately 10 million American adults annually and anxiety affecting almost twice that number (W.E. Narrow, unpublished data, July 1998;

W.E. Narrow, D.S. Rae, and D.A. Regier, unpublished data, July 1998).

In this chapter, we review the recent evidence linking cardiovascular disease and depression and anxiety; the neuropsychiatric and psychological effects of high-technology cardiac care; the psychiatric syndromes that present with cardiac symptoms; the neuropsychiatric toxicity of cardiac drugs; and the cardiovascular side effects of psychotropic medications.

Historical Perspective

Early studies estimated the co-occurrence of depression and CAD as 18%–60%; more recent studies have narrowed the estimates to 16%–23% (Musselman et al. 1998). Accumulated evidence suggests that this significant overlap between depression and CAD is not merely an artifact of the predictable co-occurrence of two highly prevalent conditions but rather an indication of genuine "two-way connections" between psychiatric disorders and cardiovascular disease (Shapiro 1996). Similar bidirectional links between anxiety, and possibly other psychiatric disorders, and CAD also may exist.

The interplay between psychiatric disorders and cardiac disease has been the subject of several recent reviews, to which the interested reader is referred (Glassman and Shapiro 1998; Januzzi et al. 2000; Musselman et al. 1998; Shapiro 1996). Suffice it to say that depression appears to be an independent risk factor for the development and progression of CAD, and the combination of depression and CAD portends greater morbidity and mortality than does either one alone (Frasure-Smith et al. 1993, 1995). Even in patients without preexisting heart disease, depression heightens the risk for cardiac mortality (Penninx et al. 2001). Moreover, when the full armamentarium of high-technology cardiac care—permanent pacemakers, automatic internal cardioverter defibrillators (AICDs), left ventricular assist devices (LVADs), cardiac allotransplantation—is used, patients experience a panoply of neuropsychiatric effects and psychosocial crises.

Putative mediators of the inferior outcomes in patients with the combination of CAD and depression or anxiety have been recently reviewed (Glassman and Shapiro 1998; Januzzi et al. 2000; Musselman et al. 1998) and include

- A hyperactive hypothalamic-pituitary-adrenocortical axis
- An excess of circulating catecholamines
- An exaggerated response to stress
- A state of greater platelet aggregability
- An alteration in lipid metabolism
- An alteration in cardiac rhythm
- A diminution in heart rate variability

Based on their study of more than 88,000 elderly Medicare recipients with myocardial infarction (MI), Druss and his colleagues (2001) advanced the disturbing hypothesis that differences in the quality of medical care received by patients with cardiac and psychiatric disorders and by cardiac patients without comorbid psychiatric illness may explain the higher rates of cardiac mortality in the former group. Differences in the use of various interventions after MI (e.g., reperfusion therapy) were largely seen in patients for whom the benefit of such treatments was equivocal.

Psychiatric Disorders in Patients With Transplants and Implantable Devices

Ample evidence implicates depression and anxiety as contributory factors in the occurrence and progression of CAD. What, then, of the other arrow in the bidirectional link between psychiatric disorders and heart disease? In this section, we examine the psychological ramifications and psychiatric complications of four major cardiac interventions: permanent pacemakers, AICDs, LVADs, and cardiac allotransplantation.

Permanent Pacemakers

Within a decade of the first use of permanent pacemakers in the late 1950s, psychiatric investigators had already begun to chart the course of patients' psychological reactions to these devices.

One early study (Blacher and Basch 1970) was interesting, not only for its contribution to our understanding of the post-pace-maker-implantation course but also for its descriptive approach to psychopathology and for its inclusion of verbatim patient comments.

According to these researchers, patients progress over time through three characteristic phases of response following pace-maker implantation. In the first phase (the perioperative phase), patients are understandably preoccupied with the prospect of surgery involving the heart; the implications of an unsuccessful operative procedure; and the need to relinquish control of a vital bodily function to an artificial, battery-powered device. Patients' comments (e.g., "I'm a mechanic, and I know that machines break down, but not this machine") during this initial phase si-multaneously captured both their awareness and their denial of this precarious dependence on a machine.

In the middle phase (the adaptive phase), when individuals are postimplantation and out of the hospital, patients feel free from danger and begin to incorporate the device into their lives and self-representations. As demonstrated by one patient who actually anthropomorphized the pacemaker, the device was psy-chologically internalized (much as a relationship with a signifi-cant other is): "After a while, we got used to each other, and I didn't notice it anymore." If depression was to complicate the postimplantation course, it emerged in this middle phase and oc-curred in 12 of the 50 subjects in this study.

In the final phase (the long-range phase), comments from pa-tients who remained ambivalent about the device suggested that they viewed it as an internalized (literally) bad object: "If only they could find a way to treat the heart and take this thing out." Another patient queried, "Why do I need a thing like this hang-ing on me?" However, most patients made an adequate adjust-ment to the implanted device. Indeed, in another study, nearly half of the patients adjusted to the device in less than 1 month (Duru et al. 2001).

Another modern investigation, which relied on validated di-agnostic criteria, studied 84 patients between 15 days and more than 2 years after implantation; a point prevalence of 19% was found for psychiatric disorders (Aydemir et al. 1997). Not surprisingly, diagnoses were primarily adjustment, depressive, and anxiety disorders; the most frequent symptoms included difficulties at work and with activities, anxiety, anergia, hypochondriasis, and insomnia. However, because of lack of a control group and of premorbid psychiatric information, one cannot impute causality to the implanted pacemaker.

Duru et al. (2001) found a rate of probable anxiety of 13.1%; depressive disorders were found in 5.2% of the patients. In an interesting comparison, these rates were statistically identical to those in patients with AICDs.

Automatic Internal Cardioverter Defibrillators

First used in 1980, AICDs are implantable, battery-operated devices that function similarly to permanent pacemakers; they sense the cardiac rhythm and electrically shock the heart to terminate potentially fatal ventricular tachyarrhythmias. Each discharge applies 25 or 30 joules and lasts between 3 and 8 seconds (Pycha et al. 1986). These devices are a boon to those patients whose arrhythmias have proven refractory to medical management. However, in an ultimate experience of ambivalence, this automatic, abortive, ultimately lifesaving, electrical response simultaneously engenders apprehension in AICD patients, who live with the constant threat of being shocked while fully conscious (Heller et al. 1998). Turning a bedrock principle of operant conditioning on its head, the AICD requires patients to maintain behavior (i.e., live) despite being "punished" (i.e., shocked) for it (Keren et al. 1991).

Thus, it is not surprising that these devices should be associated with anxious and depressive symptoms and disorders. In the perioperative period, patients experience anxiety, fear, and depression amid diagnosis with a life-threatening condition, treatment with a two-phase invasive procedure, compromise of self-efficacy, and disruption of body image (Pycha et al. 1986). In the later postimplantation phase, however, abetted by a healthy, adaptive use of denial, patients nearly uniformly view the device as a source of both physical and psychological security (Pycha et al. 1986). In fact, AICD patients—even those who have been shocked—view the device as a source of security to a like degree as do patients with pacemakers (Duru et al. 2001).

Centered on the adaptive deployment of denial as a defense against the anxiety engendered by the AICD, Fricchione and his colleagues (1989) offered an intriguing conceptualization of patients' reactions to this device. Patients may react to the AICD in a fashion similar to the response of some patients to addictive anxiolytic medications; namely, they may abuse, become dependent on, and, if it is removed, experience withdrawal from the device, whereas others may react with panic-level anxiety to AICD placement. For example, discharge of the AICD may overwhelm a patient with panic and render impossible his or her efforts to deny that he or she actually has a potentially fatal arrhythmia for which the AICD was implanted in the first place. The patient who "abuses" his or her AICD endows it with an unfailing ability to save his or her life no matter how reckless and risk-laden his or her lifestyle. This patient deploys a maladaptively high amount of denial, in contrast to the AICD-dependent patient who denies the seriousness of his or her condition sparingly little and thus subjugates himself or herself to the machine. Finally, the patient whose AICD is explanted may find his or her source of denial and security removed as well; without it, his or her anxiety is left unchecked and unmanageable.

The degree of psychological disequilibrium experienced by AICD patients may be explained by the adaptiveness of the defenses deployed against it. Offering a less dynamic explanation, recent literature has suggested that psychological disruption may increase with the greater number of shocks delivered by the AICD (Heller et al. 1998; Herrmann et al. 1997). In a group of 63 AICD-treated patients (with a mean duration of AICD placement of nearly 18 months), more than half of the patients who received 10 or more shocks showed elevated scores of anxiety and depression (Herrmann et al. 1997). Not even one-tenth of the patients who had been shocked fewer than four times showed abnormal scores. In another study, compared with 30 patients who experienced no discharges, 28 patients who experienced one discharge worried more about their families and their health, reduced their participation in new activities, and were sadder (Heller et al. 1998).

It may well be that amid a shower of gunfire, it is decidedly more difficult to deny that one is in war. However, even though patients who were shocked by the AICD reported greater anxiety and more limitations in leisure activities, they nevertheless considered their device a "life extender" (Duru et al. 2001).

Left Ventricular Assist Devices

The history of the LVAD begins in 1964, when the National Heart, Lung, and Blood Institute initiated development of mechanical devices, including the total artificial heart, intended to assume the pump function of the left ventricle and thus restore end-organ (e.g., brain, kidney) perfusion (D.J. Goldstein et al. 1998). LVADs were initially bulky and noisy and precluded the patient's discharge from the hospital. Current LVADs, however, are wearable devices, powered by two rechargeable batteries and worn as a belt, vest, or holster, that permit patients not only to leave the hospital but also to lead full and productive lives (D.J. Goldstein et al. 1998). In fact, 44 of 90 recipients of a wearable LVAD were discharged successfully to resume driving, working, attending school, and engaging in recreational activities; all were either transplanted or explanted (as scheduled) (Morales et al. 2000).

Although their "wearability" has improved, implantation still requires a median sternotomy, through which cannulae are inserted into the left ventricle and the ascending aorta. The other ends of the tubes connect to a pumping device implanted below the diaphragm; transcutaneous wires connect it to the external batteries.

Although LVADs were originally devised as a "bridge to transplantation" for patients awaiting a heart transplant, and approved by the U.S. Food and Drug Administration (FDA) for this purpose in 1994, cardiac surgeons are now considering LVADs as "destination therapy" or a "bridge to recovery" (D.J. Goldstein et al. 1998; Sun et al. 1999). In fact, the Randomized Evaluation of Mechanical Assistance for the Treatment of Congestive Heart

Failure (REMATCH) trial was launched in May 1998 to investigate this indication.

Much of what we know about the use of LVADs and their psychological effects comes from clinician-investigators at Columbia Presbyterian Medical Center in New York City, the site of an active heart transplant program. Shapiro and his colleagues (1996) reported on Columbia Presbyterian's first 30 LVAD recipients. Although 40% of their cohort were free of any psychiatric disorder preoperatively, one in five patients had an acute encephalopathy or organic mental syndrome, which had been undetected by the surgical team. Not surprisingly, the presence of cognitive impairment proved to be a risk factor for postoperative neuropsychiatric disturbance, including stroke. In total, 25 of the 30 patients required psychiatric intervention after implantation; in addition to organic mental syndromes, problems included family distress; difficulty coping with prolonged hospitalization; and, most notably, five new cases of depression. These were successfully treated with psychotherapy, serotonergic antidepressants, and psychostimulants.

Cardiac Allotransplantation

Although the technique of cardiac allotransplantation has changed little since Barnard performed the first human-to-human heart transplant more than 30 years ago, the availability of immunosuppressive agents in the 1980s resulted in improved survival rates for heart transplant recipients (S.A. Hunt 1998). Nonetheless, rejection, opportunistic infections, and the development of coronary arteriopathy in the transplanted heart remain problematic (S.A. Hunt 1998). Psychologically, the entire undertaking is rife with opportunity for psychosocial disequilibrium and neuropsychiatric disturbance. It is useful to consider separately the various phases of the transplant process and their attendant psychiatric, psychological, and social complications.

Prelisting Psychiatric Evaluation and Waiting Period

Psychiatric evaluation is generally required before a patient can be listed as a heart-transplant candidate. Adjustment disorders, anxiety, and depression are routinely observed. Attributed to the seriousness of the underlying medical condition, these conditions do not necessarily contraindicate transplant candidacy (Freeman et al. 1988; Kuhn et al. 1988; Mai 1993; Shapiro and Kornfeld 1989). Not surprisingly, patients who present management problems for the transplant team during this early phase are found to have personality disorders, substance abuse, dementia, delirium, and somatization disorder; these problems tend to persist throughout the entire transplantation course (Kuhn et al. 1988). Antisocial, histrionic, dependent, and passive-aggressive personality traits; substance abuse; past or current depression; and noncompliance with prior medical regimens may heighten risk for noncompliance, perioperative morbidity, and even mortality (Freeman et al. 1988; Shapiro et al. 1995).

After being listed as a candidate, the patient must wait for a donor heart, fully appreciating that another family will pay dearly for his or her benefit. Understandably, anxiety and depression continue into this phase of anticipation (Kuhn et al. 1988; Mai 1993).

Postoperative Period

The hallmark of the postoperative period, transient confusion, may be related to the use of steroids to prevent rejection or to a metabolic encephalopathy; it uniformly appears early after surgery (Freeman et al. 1988; Kuhn et al. 1988; Shapiro and Kornfeld 1989). Also prominent in this period are affective disturbances, both manic and depressive. Depression can be related to a protracted hospitalization posttransplant or to steroid use, whereas hypomanic symptoms tend to remit with a steroid taper (Shapiro and Kornfeld 1989).

Once the patient has fully recovered from the operation, he or she awakens to the realization that perhaps his or her most vital organ has been replaced by a foreign object, indeed one that has been removed from someone, unknown to him or her, who has died (Mai 1993). Some patients deny the significance of this momentous event, whereas others experience guilt, anxiety, and even fear that the transplanted heart will somehow alter their native personality (Kuhn et al. 1988; Mai 1993).

Long Range

Behaviorally disturbed patients may fare particularly poorly over the long term (Freeman et al. 1988; Kuhn et al. 1988). Of five patients with persistent behavior problems, one died due to addiction-related noncompliance, one became noncompliant as a result of depression, and one required repeated psychiatric hospitalization for suicidal behavior (Kuhn et al. 1988). Another patient (who was considered at the prelisting evaluation to have narcissistic and potentially antisocial personality traits) died after missing a clinic appointment; he arrived later in acute rejection, a condition thought to be associated with alcohol-related noncompliance (Shapiro and Kornfeld 1989).

Financial worries, marital discord, family conflicts, and sexual dysfunction also dominate this phase, although these issues tend to diminish after 12–18 months (Shapiro and Kornfeld 1989). Over the long term, most transplanted patients fare well in all domains, despite the enormity of the physical and psychological tolls imposed by cardiac transplantation.

Psychiatric Disorders That Present With Cardiac Symptoms

Several psychiatric syndromes may either cause cardiac symptoms or lead patients to attribute psychic distress to a cardiovascular disorder. In fact, numerous reports document a relatively high prevalence of hypochondriasis, somatization, anxiety, and depression in patients who complain of chest pain but do not have significant CAD (Bass and Wade 1984; Channer et al. 1985; McLaurin et al. 1977; Ostfeld et al. 1964; Wielgosz et al. 1984). In addition, patients with psychogenic pain disorder, factitious disorder, and complex partial seizures may initially present to an internist or a cardiologist with various cardiovascular complaints (Tesar and Stern 1989).

Anxiety and Mood Disorders

About 20 million American adults between ages 18 and 54 have an anxiety disorder; many have comorbid depression (W.E. Narrow,

D.S. Rae, D.A. Regier, unpublished data July 1998). Among these individuals, symptoms of panic and generalized anxiety are frequently associated with cardiorespiratory symptoms and signs, some of which are even codified in diagnostic criteria (e.g., chest discomfort, shortness of breath, palpitations, tachycardia). Several colorful names have been applied over the decades to those patients with anxiety disorders with cardiac symptomatology: neurocirculatory asthenia, hyperkinetic heart syndrome, essential circulatory hyperkinesis, hyperventilation syndrome, and hyperdynamic β-adrenergic circulatory state (Frohlich et al. 1969; Wheeler 1966). Whatever the label, these patients frequently are the subjects of extensive cardiac evaluations and invasive diagnostic procedures before an accurate psychiatric diagnosis is made.

A variety of clinically insignificant bodily sensations tend to preoccupy the minds of some patients with depression, even those without anxiety. Such rumination may amplify the experience of the particular sensation and, in some cases, may spawn actual physical abnormalities (e.g., tachycardia, diaphoresis).

Somatoform Disorders

Somatization disorder, hypochondriasis, and pain disorder share common features. They include persistent complaints or fears of symptoms that suggest physical illness in the absence of an explanatory pathophysiological mechanism but occur in association with a presumed or identified psychological conflict. In the case of pain disorder, a physical basis to the pain may be identified, but the pain is thought to be disproportionate to actual physical findings. These patients may repeatedly present to their primary care physicians or to emergency departments complaining of any number of cardiac symptoms. Only after several visits, and usually several diagnostic tests, does it become clear that the etiology is most likely psychological. Clinical care becomes even more difficult when patients have both a somatoform disorder and a genuine cardiac problem.

Complex Partial Seizures

Experiences of psychic phenomena (e.g., olfactory and gustatory hallucinations, micropsia, macropsia, and religious preoccupation) are well-known manifestations of complex partial seizures. Less appreciated, however, is the production of cardiovascular symptomatology (e.g., chest pain, brady- and tachyarrhythmias, and syncope) as a result of nonconvulsive electrical hyperactivity in the brain (Constantin et al. 1990; Devinsky et al. 1986; Kiok et al. 1986).

Neuropsychiatric Side Effects of Cardiovascular Medications

In addition to the various high-technology devices discussed earlier in this chapter, cardiologists, cardiac surgeons, and their patients have a vast armamentarium of pharmaceutical agents at their disposal. Case reports and small case series have documented the neuropsychiatric effects of most of these agents. Adverse consequences vary from infrequent to fairly common, but—to our knowledge—no systematic, controlled study of this adverse risk profile has ever been undertaken with sufficient methodological rigor to produce meaningful conclusions (Rauch et al. 1991).

An extensive review of the largely anecdotal literature on the neuropsychiatric adverse effects of antihypertensive medications documented the occurrence of a wide array of psychiatric symptoms and syndromes (including delirium, depression, psychosis, anxiety, fatigue, and insomnia) with the use of these agents (Rauch et al. 1991). However, the authors hastened to point out that the selection of an appropriate antihypertensive agent should be guided by common sense and by empirical evaluation on an individual basis. This advice probably applies equally to selection of medications in other classes of the cardiac pharmacopoeia.

Cardiovascular Side Effects of Psychotropic Medications

Neuroleptics

The FDA's rejection of sertindole in 1998 and the agency's requirement for a bolded warning in product information about ziprasidone—because of concern about QT prolongation with

---

both of these new atypical antipsychotics—have sparked renewed interest in the cardiovascular effects of neuroleptics. This rekindled interest in the QT interval merits a brief discussion of its physiology and measurement.

The QT interval is the electrocardiographic representation of ventricular depolarization and subsequent repolarization; it is measured from the beginning of the Q wave to the end of the T wave. Because this interval varies with heart rate (the faster the heart rate, the shorter the QT interval), correction for this parameter is required. The most widely used formula for this correction is Bazett's formula, resulting in the corrected QT interval (QT_c)

$$QT_c = QT \div \sqrt{RR}$$

where RR is the interval between the two R waves preceding the measured QT interval. In our experience, electrocardiogram (ECG) machines routinely overestimate the QT_c, likely because they mistake the U for the T wave. Thus, we recommend that the QT_c be measured and calculated by hand, preferably in lead II, but practically in whichever lead yields a well-defined T wave.

Prolongation of the QT interval is associated with a potentially fatal ventricular tachyarrhythmia called *torsades de pointes*, named for its characteristic ECG pattern resembling a twisting of points. However, the relation between QT prolongation and cardiac arrhythmia is complicated by several factors (N. Hunt and Stern 1995; Welch and Chue 2000):

- The normal duration of the QT interval has not been definitively established.
- The so-called critical QT interval at which risk of arrhythmia is greatest is unknown.
- The QT_c can be prolonged without causing torsades de pointes.
- Torsades de pointes can occur even when the QT_c is normal.
- Torsades de pointes occurs in only a minority of patients with a lengthened QT_c.
- Other risk factors for torsades de pointes include hypokalemia, hypocalcemia, and hypomagnesemia.

Sertindole and ziprasidone were not the first neuroleptic medications to be associated with QT prolongation; the phenothiazines, pimozide, and haloperidol also have been implicated. In fact, some of the older, conventional neuroleptics are significantly more cardiotoxic than the newer agents and might well fall short of current cardiac safety standards (Welch and Chue 2000). Haloperidol, because of its widespread use in intravenous form in hospitalized, medically ill patients who may be at particular risk to develop cardiac arrhythmias, has come under considerable research scrutiny. Many an indicting finger has been pointed at haloperidol when the QT_c lengthens. Reviewing this literature and citing their experience with the use of large doses of intravenous haloperidol in medically compromised patients, N. Hunt and Stern (1995) concluded that the use of intravenous haloperidol is rarely an independent cause of torsades de pointes. A recent study found a statistically significant difference in average change in QT_c between groups treated with intravenous haloperidol and groups not treated with intravenous haloperidol, but the difference was not clinically significant (having increased from 445 msec to only 454 msec) (Hatta et al. 2001). Even when the QT_c was prolonged by more than 100 msec in two patients, neither had an arrhythmia.

In our clinical practice, intravenous haloperidol has been used safely to treat acutely agitated, delirious, medically ill patients (including those with cardiac disease); we refrain from its use or discontinue the agent only when the QT_c is 500 msec or greater or increases beyond 25% from an individual's baseline. We monitor serum levels of potassium, magnesium, and calcium; replenish these electrolytes when necessary; and interpret the appearance of U waves and flattened T waves on the ECG as evidence of incipient arrhythmia.

Five so-called atypical antipsychotics are now available in the United States: clozapine, risperidone, olanzapine, quetiapine, and ziprasidone. Although these agents are less likely than older agents to cause extrapyramidal side effects, as a group their adverse effects on weight, glucose regulation, and lipid metabolism have been increasingly recognized (including an association with type 2 diabetes mellitus presenting as diabetic ketoacidosis) (L. E. Goldstein et al. 1999).

Antidepressant Agents

Tricyclic Antidepressants

Tricyclic antidepressants (TCAs) are well known to have cardio-vascular and autonomic side effects, including orthostatic hypotension, tachycardia and other anticholinergic effects, and cardiac conduction delays.

Postural hypotension, resulting primarily from blockade of α_1-adrenergic receptors, can result in falls, which may lead to fractures, head injury, and, for patients taking anticoagulants, bleeding. It can occur with any of the TCAs, even with small doses, but is more common with the tertiary amines (e.g., amitriptyline, imipramine) than with the secondary amines (e.g., nortriptyline, protriptyline). Although desipramine is a secondary amine, its potential to cause orthostatic hypotension is similar to that of its parent compound, imipramine.

Anticholinergic effects of these medications, including dry mouth, blurred vision, urinary hesitancy, and constipation, are frequently the cause of patient discomfort and thus discontinuation of TCAs. Tachycardia, agitation, and delirium may eventuate with anticholinergic toxicity. In cardiac patients, these outcomes can be particularly problematic; they may result in excess myocardial demand, arrhythmia, and the dislodging or outright removal of various pieces of critical equipment (e.g., an intra-aortic balloon pump).

The TCAs prolong the PR, QRS, and QT intervals, thus rendering these agents potentially proarrhythmic and, therefore, dangerous in overdose (Stern et al. 1985). However, they also possess effects similar to those of class IA antiarrhythmics, such as quinidine, and thus may be safe in, if not beneficial to, patients with cardiac rhythm disturbances. However, data from the Cardiac Arrhythmia Suppression Trials I and II significantly altered cardiologists' views on the benefit of antiarrhythmic therapy in the immediate post-MI period (Glassman et al. 1993, 1998). These studies found that encainide and flecainide, both class IC antiarrhythmics, and moricizine, a class IA agent, increased mortality in post-MI patients. Therefore, TCAs may be similarly dangerous in MI patients and, by extrapolation, may be harmful to patients with cardiac disease in general. Fortunately, newer agents are available, not only with theoretical advantages in cardiac patients but also with emerging research evidence of their cardiac safety.

Selective Serotonin Reuptake Inhibitors

In the United States, five selective serotonin reuptake inhibitors (SSRIs) are available: fluoxetine, sertraline, paroxetine, fluvoxamine, and citalopram. Although heart rate may slow moderately with their use, these agents are not known to affect appreciably cardiac conduction or blood pressure, either supine or standing, even in patients with heart disease. In an open-label, 7-week study of fluoxetine in 27 depressed patients with heart disease, this SSRI appeared to be safe (with no significant change in heart rate, blood pressure, or cardiac conduction) (Roose et al. 1998a). Similarly, in a randomized, double-blind, 6-week study of paroxetine and nortriptyline in 81 patients with depression and ischemic heart disease, the SSRI effected no persistent change in cardiac rhythm, heart rate, or heart rate variability (Roose et al. 1998b). Still, the authors of both studies cautioned against a sweeping assertion of safety of SSRIs in cardiac patients on the basis of these two small studies of limited duration.

Even in patients after MI, SSRIs appear to be safe. The first study of SSRI therapy in the post-MI population, the Sertraline Anti-Depressant Heart Attack Trial, was an open-label, 16-week study of sertraline in 26 patients with depression 5–30 days after MI (Shapiro et al. 1999). Similar to the studies of fluoxetine and paroxetine in cardiac patients without MI, sertraline was found to exert no significant effect on heart rate, blood pressure, cardiac conduction, ejection fraction, or coagulation measures. These investigators subsequently launched a randomized, placebo-controlled trial of sertraline in depressed post-MI patients.

Mood Stabilizers

Rather than cardiovascular toxicities, the side-effect profiles of lithium, carbamazepine, and valproate—the three major mood stabilizers—are dominated by adverse reactions affecting other organ systems, primarily hematological, hepatic, and dermatological. Despite this relative cardiovascular safety, a few points warrant brief mention.

Lithium may cause flattening or inversion of T waves that is generally inconsequential and reversible on discontinuation of lithium. Because of the occurrence of sinoatrial node dysfunction in some lithium-treated patients, patients with preexisting sick sinus syndrome may require a permanent pacemaker before lithium therapy can be safely initiated. Cases of atrial and ventricular arrhythmias have been sporadically reported at therapeutic serum levels, although these disturbances are more common in cases of lithium toxicity. In states of relative sodium deficit, the kidney will attempt to reabsorb sodium. Because of its similarity to sodium, lithium, too, will be reclaimed in these situations, and toxicity may eventuate. Thus, treatment with a low-sodium diet, thiazide diuretics, or angiotensin-converting enzyme (ACE) inhibitors may elevate the serum lithium level.

Structurally similar to imipramine, carbamazepine, like TCAs, may cause cardiac conduction delay. By virtue of hepatic enzyme induction, carbamazepine may diminish the effectiveness of warfarin. Neurotoxic effects of carbamazepine may be more likely when it is combined with ACE inhibitors or calcium channel blockers.

Valproate appears to be free of any adverse cardiac effect.

Summary

Regardless of practice venue, psychiatrists frequently see patients with both psychiatric and cardiac illnesses. Not merely an artifact of the high prevalence of these disorders in the American populace, the frequent comorbidity of diseases of the mind and the heart is evidence of the reciprocal relation between the two. Both etiologically and therapeutically, one has effects on the other; knowledge of these bidirectional links is imperative for any psychiatrist. With an increasing proportion of patients undergoing LVAD and AICD implantation—and with the development of high-technology cardiac treatments of ever greater sophistication—psychiatrists can expect to see the myriad of psychological and neuropsychiatric effects of cardiac disease and its treatment well into the next decade and beyond.

References

Aydemir Ö, Özmen E, Küey L, et al: Psychiatric morbidity and depressive symptomatology in patients with permanent pacemakers. Pacing and Clinical Electrophysiology 20:1628–1632, 1997

Bass C, Wade C: Chest pain with normal coronary arteries: a comparative study of psychiatric and social morbidity. Psychol Med 14:51–61, 1984

Blacher RS, Basch SH: Psychological aspects of pacemaker implantation. Arch Gen Psychiatry 22:319–323, 1970

Centers for Disease Control and Prevention and American Heart Association: National Health and Nutrition Examination Survey III, 1988–1994. Hyattsville, MD, Centers for Disease Control and Prevention and American Heart Association, 1996

Channer KS, James MA, Papouchado M, et al: Anxiety and depression in patients with chest pain referred for exercise testing. Lancet 2:820–823, 1985

Constantin L, Martins JB, Fincham RW, et al: Bradycardia and syncope as manifestations of partial epilepsy. J Am Coll Cardiol 15:900–905, 1990

Devinsky O, Price BH, Cohen SI: Cardiac manifestations of complex partial seizures. Am J Med 80:195–202, 1986

Druss BG, Bradford WD, Rosenheck RA, et al: Quality of medical care and excess mortality in older patients with mental disorders. Arch Gen Psychiatry 58:565–572, 2001

Duru F, Büchi S, Klaghofer R, et al: How different from pacemaker patients are recipients of implantable cardioverter-defibrillators with respect to psychosocial adaptation, affective disorders, and quality of life? Heart 85:375–379, 2001

Frasure-Smith N, Lespérance F, Talajic M: Depression following myocardial infarction: impact on 6-month survival. JAMA 270:1819–1825, 1993

Frasure-Smith N, Lespérance F, Talajic M: Depression and 18-month prognosis after myocardial infarction. Circulation 91:999–1005, 1995

Freeman AM, Folks DG, Sokol RS, et al: Cardiac transplantation: clinical correlates of psychiatric outcome. Psychosomatics 29:47–54, 1988

Fricchione GL, Olson LC, Vlay SC: Psychiatric syndromes in patients with the automatic internal cardioverter defibrillator: anxiety, psychological dependence, abuse, and withdrawal. Am Heart J 117: 1411–1414, 1989

Frohlich ED, Tarazi RC, Dustan HP: Hyperdynamic beta-adrenergic circulatory state: increased beta-receptor responsiveness. Arch Intern Med 123:1–7, 1969

Glassman AH, Shapiro PA: Depression and the course of coronary artery disease. Am J Psychiatry 155:4–11, 1998

Glassman AH, Roose SP, Bigger JT: The safety of tricyclic antidepressants in cardiac patients: risk-benefit reconsidered. JAMA 269:2673–2675, 1993

Glassman AH, Rodriguez AI, Shapiro PA: The use of antidepressant drugs in patients with heart disease. J Clin Psychiatry 59 (suppl 10):16–21, 1998

Goldstein DJ, Oz MC, Rose EA: Implantable left ventricular assist devices. N Engl J Med 339:1522–1533, 1998

Goldstein LE, Sporn J, Brown S, et al: New-onset diabetes mellitus and diabetic ketoacidosis associated with olanzapine treatment. Psychosomatics 40:438–443, 1999

Hatta K, Takahashi T, Nakamura H, et al: The association between intravenous haloperidol and prolonged QT interval. J Clin Psychopharmacol 21:257–261, 2001

Heller SS, Ormont MA, Lidagoster L, et al: Psychosocial outcome after ICD implantation: a current perspective. Pacing and Clinical Electrophysiology 21:1207–1215, 1998

Herrmann C, Von Zur Mühen F, Schaumann A, et al: Standardized assessment of psychological well-being and quality-of-life in patients with implanted defibrillators. Pacing and Clinical Electrophysiology 20(part 1):95–103, 1997

Hunt N, Stern TA: The association between intravenous haloperidol and torsades de pointes. Psychosomatics 36:541–549, 1995

Hunt SA: Current status of cardiac transplantation. JAMA 280:1692–1698, 1998

Januzzi JL, Stern TA, Pasternak RC, et al: The influence of anxiety and depression on outcomes of patients with coronary artery disease. Arch Intern Med 160:1913–1921, 2000

Keren R, Aarons D, Veltri EP: Anxiety and depression in patients with life-threatening ventricular arrhythmias: impact of the implantable cardioverter-defibrillator. Pacing and Clinical Electrophysiology 14:181–187, 1991

Kiok MC, Terrence CF, Fromm GH, et al: Sinus arrest in epilepsy. Neurology 36:115–116, 1986

Kuhn WF, Myers B, Brennan AF, et al: Psychopathology in heart transplant candidates. Journal of Heart Transplantation 7:223–226, 1988

Mai FM: Psychiatric aspects of heart transplantation. Br J Psychiatry 163:285–292, 1993

McLaurin LP, Raft D, Tate SC: Chest pain with normal coronaries: a psychosomatic illness? Circulation 56 (suppl 3):174, 1977

Morales DLS, Catanese KA, Helman DN, et al: Six-year experience of caring for forty-four patients with a left ventricular assist device at home: safe, economical, necessary. J Thorac Cardiovasc Surg 119: 251–259, 2000

Musselman DL, Evans DL, Nemeroff CB: The relationship of depression to cardiovascular disease: epidemiology, biology, and treatment. Arch Gen Psychiatry 55:580–592, 1998

Ostfeld AM, Lebovits BZ, Shekelle RB, et al: A prospective study of the relationship between personality and coronary heart disease. Journal of Chronic Diseases 17:265–276, 1964

Penninx BWJH, Beekman ATF, Honig A, et al: Depression and cardiac mortality: results from a community-based longitudinal study. Arch Gen Psychiatry 58:221–227, 2001

Pycha C, Gulledge AD, Hutzler J, et al: Psychological responses to the implantable defibrillator: preliminary observations. Psychosomatics 27:841–845, 1986

Rauch SL, Stern TA, Zusman RM: Neuropsychiatric considerations in the treatment of hypertension. Int J Psychiatry Med 21:291–308, 1991

Roose SP, Glassman AH, Attia E, et al: Cardiovascular effects of fluoxetine in depressed patients with heart disease. Am J Psychiatry 155:660–665, 1998a

Roose SP, Laghrissi-Thode F, Kennedy JS, et al: Comparison of paroxetine and nortriptyline in depressed patients with ischemic heart disease. JAMA 279:287–291, 1998b

Shapiro PA: Psychiatric aspects of cardiovascular disease. Psychiatr Clin North Am 19:613–629, 1996

Shapiro PA, Kornfeld DS: Psychiatric outcome of heart transplantation. Gen Hosp Psychiatry 11:352–357, 1989

Shapiro PA, Williams DL, Foray AT: Psychosocial evaluation and prediction of compliance problems and morbidity after heart transplantation. Transplantation 60:1462–1466, 1995

Shapiro PA, Levin HR, Oz MC: Left ventricular assist devices: psychosocial burden and implications for heart transplant programs. Gen Hosp Psychiatry 18:30S–35S, 1996

Shapiro PA, Lespérance F, Frasure-Smith N, et al: An open-label preliminary trial of sertraline for treatment of major depression after acute myocardial infarction (the SADHAT trial). Am Heart J 137:1100–1106, 1999

Stern TA, O'Gara PT, Mulley AG, et al: Complications after overdose with tricyclic antidepressants. Crit Care Med 13:672–674, 1985

Sun BC, Catanese KA, Spanier TB, et al: 100 Long-term implantable left ventricular assist devices: the Columbia Presbyterian interim experience. Ann Thorac Surg 68:688–694, 1999

Tesar GE, Stern TA: Psychiatric issues in the cardiac patient, in The Practice of Cardiology, 2nd Edition. Edited by Eagle KA, Haber E, DeSanctis RW, et al. Boston, MA, Little, Brown, 1989, pp 1759–1790

Welch R, Chue P: Antipsychotic agents and QT changes. J Psychiatry Neurosci 25:154–160, 2000

Wheeler EO: Emotional stress: Cardiovascular disease, cardiovascular symptoms, and emotional stress, in The Heart, Arteries, and Veins. Edited by Hurst JW, Logue RB. New York, McGraw-Hill, 1966, pp 1106–1116

Wielgosz AT, Fletcher RH, McCants CB, et al: Unimproved chest pain in patients with minimal or no coronary disease: a behavioral phenomenon. Am Heart J 108:67–72, 1984

Chapter 2

Psychiatric Aspects of Gastroenterology

Steven A. Epstein, M.D.
Ahmed Sherif Meguid, M.B., Ch.B.
Thomas N. Wise, M.D.

The gastrointestinal system and the mind are closely inter-twined. In recent years, well-designed research has begun to elu-cidate the complex area of brain-gut interactions. Comorbidity between psychiatric disorders and certain functional bowel dis-orders also has been clearly established (see Drossman et al. 1999 for an excellent recent review). Behavior problems such as alco-hol abuse clearly lead to gastrointestinal disorders such as cirrho-sis. Because of these and other factors, a significant proportion of a gastroenterologist's clinical activities may be focused on symp-toms that are affected by psychological factors. In this chapter, we highlight areas of importance for psychiatrists as they relate to organs of the gastrointestinal system.

Esophageal Disorders

Gastroesophageal Reflux Disease

Gastroesophageal reflux disease (GERD) is a general term used to describe the clinical consequences of reflux of stomach and

---

This chapter is in part an updated and expanded version of Epstein SA, Randel LB, Wise TN: "Gastroenterology," in *Psychiatric Care of the Medical Patient*, 2nd Edition. Edited by Stoudemire A, Fogel BS, Greenberg D. New York, Oxford University Press, 2000.

duodenal contents into the esophagus. Patients with GERD usually present with acid regurgitation, heartburn, and dysphagia. It is also the most common cause of noncardiac chest pain. GERD may be caused by reflux (due to decreased lower esophageal sphincter pressure, a motility disorder [see "Esophageal Motility Disorders" below]), decreased esophageal clearance (e.g., from anticholinergic medications), and increased gastric acid. Evaluation and treatment should consist of a complete history, endoscopy, and an empirical trial of an antireflux medication (e.g., omeprazole) (Kahrilas 1998). However, it is important to realize that mild, uncomplicated heartburn is quite common; more than 10% of adult Americans experience heartburn at least weekly (Kahrilas 1998). Chronic GERD may lead to Barrett's esophagus, in which the healing epithelium is replaced by specialized columnar epithelium with intestinal metaplasia, a precursor of esophageal cancer (Cohen and Parkman 2000).

Treatment of reflux begins with conservative measures: avoiding late-night snacks and lying down after meals; elevating the head of the bed; reducing intake of fatty foods, chocolate, alcohol, and cigarettes; and taking antacids as needed (Katz 1995a). Anticholinergic agents such as tertiary amine tricyclic antidepressants (TCAs) and low-potency neuroleptics should be avoided if possible. If the above measures fail, histamine-2 (H_2) receptor antagonists (e.g., ranitidine) or proton pump inhibitors (e.g., omeprazole) may be used. Proton pump inhibitors are more efficacious than H_2 blockers, although the latter are more widely used (Kahrilas 1998).

Reflux also may be treated with promotility drugs such as bethanechol and metoclopramide. Metoclopramide appears to sensitize tissues to acetylcholine, thereby increasing lower esophageal sphincter pressure and increasing gastric emptying. Its antiemetic properties are due to its antagonism of dopamine-2 receptors. Pharmacological effects generally last for 1–2 hours. Approximately 10% of the patients who are regularly prescribed metoclopramide experience restlessness, drowsiness, and fatigue. According to the Reglan package insert (A.H. Robins), extrapyramidal symptoms may occur in 1 in 500 patients and usually are dystonic reactions (see Table 2–1). Extrapyramidal symptoms are particularly common in elderly patients and patients with renal failure because the drug is predominantly renally excreted. There have been reports of depression and other psychiatric disturbances as well. Because of these problems, as well as its generally low efficacy, metoclopramide is not a good choice for patients with GERD (Kahrilas 1998). If metoclopramide or another promotility agent (e.g., bethanechol) is unsuccessful, antireflux surgery to increase lower esophageal sphincter competence may be tried.

Table 2–1. Selected psychiatric side effects of medications used for gastrointestinal disorders

Medication	Gastrointestinal disorder	Potential psychiatric side effects
Metoclopramide	Gastroesophageal reflux disease	Extrapyramidal symptoms
Histamine-2 blockers	Peptic ulcer disease	Delirium
Corticosteroids	Inflammatory bowel disease	Insomnia, anxiety, depression, psychosis, delirium
Interferon alpha	Hepatitis B and C	Anxiety, depression, cognitive impairment; may be severe

Esophageal Motility Disorders

Normal motor functioning of the esophagus requires proper coordination of the upper esophageal sphincter, esophageal body, and lower esophageal sphincter. A motility disorder results from failure of any of these components (Cohen and Parkman 2000). Esophageal motility disorders lead to symptoms such as chest pain, difficulty swallowing solids, difficulty ingesting liquids, heartburn, and regurgitation.

Nutcracker esophagus is a common motility abnormality that may be associated with increased visceral sensitivity. Patients with nutcracker esophagus have normal peristaltic waves of excessively high amplitude. In diffuse esophageal spasm, the patient will have simultaneous repetitive contractions and other manometric abnormalities, with peristalsis only intermittently normal. Heightened emotional arousal increases respiration and swallowing rates, which may augment esophageal distress. Anxiety that increases swallowing rates thus may exacerbate esophageal disorders (Fonagu and Calloway 1986).

Although patients often report that motility disorder symptoms are triggered by psychological stressors, no clear experimental evidence indicates that psychological stress affects esophageal motility (Whitehead 1996). In this regard, the psychiatrist must be aware that noncardiac chest pain may not be simply due to panic disorder. Other etiologies need to be carefully ruled out, including GERD, visceral hypersensitivity, and achalasia (Richter 2000).

Treatments that may be effective for chest pain from esophageal motility disorders include calcium channel blockers, imipramine (Cannon et al. 1994), other antidepressants (e.g., trazodone 100–150 mg/day), and nitrates (Katz 1995a).

Functional Esophageal Disorders

The functional gastrointestinal disorders are defined as those disorders for which a structural or biochemical basis cannot be identified. They are extremely common in primary care and gastroenterology practices and often are associated with psychosocial factors. The most important recent effort to classify these disorders is the multinational effort known as Rome II (cf., Drossman et al. 1999; http://www.romecriteria.org). Many of these disorders are discussed in their respective anatomical sections throughout this chapter.

The functional esophageal disorders include globus, rumination syndrome, functional chest pain of presumed esophageal origin, functional heartburn, and functional dysphagia. Globus is a sensation of a lump, tightness, or something stuck in the throat. It may be associated with anxiety, depression, and life stressors (Clouse et al. 1999). The older term *globus hystericus* is no longer in favor.

Rumination syndrome refers to regurgitation of food with subsequent remastication. It occurs most commonly in mentally disabled children and adults (Clouse et al. 1999). Functional chest pain of presumed esophageal origin is diagnosed when a patient has midline chest pain that is not burning. Reflux, achalasia, and other motility disorders must be ruled out. These patients have lower pain thresholds and tend to have lower standards for judging esophageal distention stimuli to be painful (Clouse et al. 1999). These psychophysiological phenomena are similar to those of irritable bowel syndrome (IBS). Treatments that help the motility disorders (e.g., low-dose antidepressants) may be helpful. Psychological treatments such as cognitive-behavioral therapy also can be useful (Ringel and Drossman 1999).

Functional heartburn is retrosternal burning discomfort in the absence of GERD. Functional dysphagia is diagnosed when the patient has a sense of solids or liquids sticking in the esophagus in the absence of GERD or a motility disorder. Psychological correlates of these conditions are not well understood (Clouse et al. 1999).

Peptic Ulcer Disease

Peptic ulcers may be gastric or duodenal. The most common contributing factors are *Helicobacter pylori* and nonsteroidal anti-inflammatory medications. Uncommon causes of relevance to psychiatrists include crack cocaine–induced perforations, presumably due to mucosal vasoconstriction. Other risk factors include having a first-degree relative with duodenal ulcer and cigarette smoking (Katz 1995b). No clear data show that specific foods or coffee consumption causes or exacerbates peptic ulcers. Similarly, although alcohol may damage the gastric mucosa, no evidence suggests that it causes peptic ulcer disease or interferes with healing (Soll 1998).

H. pylori, a gram-negative spiral organism, is probably the most common cause of both gastric and duodenal ulcers. Although 40%–60% of the population has *H. pylori* within their gastrointestinal lining, only 10%–20% of such individuals have associated disease states such as peptic ulcer disease or gastric cancer (Levenstein and Kaplan 1998). *H. pylori* alone does not explain the development of ulcers because only 7% of the individuals infected with *H. pylori* develop ulcers.

Despite clear evidence that organic factors such as *H. pylori* cause peptic ulcer disease, many patients and physicians alike still believe that psychological factors are contributory causes. Animal models support the notion that emotional stressors contribute to the development and persistence of gastric ulcers (Overmier and Murison 2000). Discriminant analysis of patients with peptic ulcer disease compared with control subjects showed depression to be the best discriminator; other major factors were increased perception of the negative effect of life events (although frequency of life events themselves did not differ), number of relatives with peptic ulcer disease, and serum pepsinogen I concentration. Behavioral risk factors such as smoking, alcohol use, and aspirin use also were significantly higher in peptic ulcer disease patients. Experimentally, emotional stress has been shown to increase gastric acid secretion in patients with duodenal ulcers (Rask-Madsen et al. 1990). Levenstein and colleagues conducted a series of epidemiological studies that found that psychological stress and lowered socioeconomic status increase the risk of developing ulcer disease (e.g., Levenstein and Kaplan 1998). Thus, peptic ulcer disease appears to be mediated by psychological, behavioral, and physiological factors (Levenstein 2000). A stress-diathesis model, in which the diathesis is *H. pylori* infection and the stressors have not been fully elucidated, would be the best way to conceptualize the development of ulcer disease (Overmier and Murison 2000). One theory, as yet unproven, is that stress, anxiety, and depression could alter immune function, thereby increasing the risk of *H. pylori* colonization or *H. pylori*–associated disease processes.

Despite the potential role for behavior therapy, direct behavioral interventions for peptic ulcer disease are in an experimental stage. Relaxation training may diminish gastric acid secretion and thus provide a therapeutic rationale for these behavioral interventions. The technical difficulties and cost of such strategies, however, prevent their widespread practical application (Bassotti and Whitehead 1994). General stress management training and psychiatric treatment should nonetheless be encouraged for individuals whose peptic ulcer disease appears to be clearly exacerbated or precipitated by stress, anxiety, or depression.

Medical Treatment

It is advisable to test for *H. pylori* before instituting treatment for the infection. Testing may be performed noninvasively with serology or a breath test. If *H. pylori* testing is negative, a proton pump inhibitor or an H_2 blocker may be used. If testing is positive, treatment consists of double therapy of acid suppression and eradication of *H. pylori* infection (J. Lee and O'Morain 1997). First-line therapy consists of 7–10 days of a proton pump inhibitor (omeprazole or lansoprazole) combined with two of three antibiotics (clarithromycin, metronidazole, or amoxicillin) (Soll 1998). Clarithromycin is a cytochrome P450 3A4,5,7 inhibitor, so potential toxicity should be monitored when medications metabolized by this enzyme are used concomitantly, including alprazolam, diazepam, triazolam, trazodone, zaleplon, and zolpidem (http://www.georgetown.edu/departments/pharmacology drug interaction Web site).

The H_2 blockers cimetidine, ranitidine, famotidine, and nizatidine continue to be used as treatments for unperforated ulcer disease. These drugs control gastric acid secretion and can help the acute lesion as well as prevent ulcer relapse. Side effects of the drugs are rare in the outpatient setting but may be more common in the sick and elderly in intensive care unit settings. They include delirium and possibly depression, although depression is not well substantiated. Ranitidine and famotidine may cause confusion, possibly less frequently than cimetidine does. It is not fully clear from the existing literature whether one H_2 blocker is truly any more likely to cause confusion than any other (Soll 1998; see Table 2–1).

Cimetidine inhibits oxidative hepatic metabolism by many cytochrome P450 enzymes. Ranitidine, however, does not impair the clearance of diazepam, lorazepam, or carbamazepine. Famotidine and nizatidine also appear to be free of cytochrome P450 interactions (Katz 1995b). Dosage of H_2 blockers should be decreased in the context of renal failure. Otherwise, an increased incidence of delirium caused by these agents will result.

Omeprazole, lansoprazole, pantoprazole, rabeprazole, and esomeprazole inhibit gastric acid secretion by altering activity of H^+/K^+–adenosine triphosphatase (ATPase) (proton pump) in gastric parietal cells. They have been shown to be extremely potent in the treatment of duodenal ulcer. Omeprazole and lansoprazole are inhibitors of the cytochrome P450 isoenzyme 2C19. When either of those medications is used, caution should be exercised when prescribing medications metabolized by this enzyme (e.g., diazepam).

The antiulcer (cytoprotective) drug sucralfate is a safe and effective alternative in susceptible patients (Katz 1995b). The agent acts locally to coat and protect ulcer sites from gastric acid and has little systemic absorption. TCAs such as doxepin also possess H_2 receptor–blocking capabilities. They should not be considered primary treatment, although they may augment and work synergistically with formal medical regimens, particularly in anxious or depressed patients with high psychophysiological gastrointestinal reactivity. Finally, surgery is used to treat ulcer patients with intractable bleeding, perforation, or nonresponse to medical therapy.

Abdominal Pain, Functional Dyspepsia, and Delayed Gastric Emptying

Chronic unexplained abdominal pain is often seen in medical practice. Functional abdominal pain as defined by the Rome II criteria must last for at least 6 months and have minimal relations to physiological events (Table 2–2). The pain must lead to loss of function and not be consciously feigned. Rome II also includes an unspecified category wherein the symptoms do not meet the full criteria set for functional abdominal pain. Before attributing abdominal pain to psychological origins, however, organic or anatomical etiologies that may have been overlooked in the initial medical evaluation must be ruled out. Acute intermittent porphyria, for example, presents with a history of chronic abdominal pain (often with a record of multiple negative exploratory laparotomies), peripheral neuropathy, and delirium. Occult intestinal adhesions also should be considered, as well as occult endometriosis in women, in whom the boundaries between abdominal and pelvic pain syndromes are blurred.

Table 2–2.   Rome II criteria for functional abdominal pain

At least 6 months of
1. Continuous or nearly continuous abdominal pain; and
2. No or only occasional relation of pain with physiological events; and
3. Some loss of daily functioning; and
4. Pain that is not feigned
5. Insufficient criteria for other functional gastrointestinal disorders that would explain the abdominal pain

---

Source.   Reprinted from Thompson WG, Longstreth GF, Drossman DA, et al: "Functional Bowel Disorders and Functional Abdominal Pain." *Gut* 45(suppl II):II43–II47, 1999. Copyright 1999 by BMJ Publishing Group. Used with permission.

The gastrointestinal discomfort in functional abdominal pain syndrome is usually described in very emotional terms or in a manner that is anatomically unusual. Jenkins (1991) found that patients with such complaints often have had a previous psychiatric disorder and that the onset of pain concurred with negative life events. Like patients with IBS, sexual abuse histories are common in patients with functional abdominal pain (Drossman et al. 1990). The increasingly recognized association between such pain syndromes and sexual abuse further suggests the need for the clinician to investigate life events and prior experiences of sexual abuse that may be associated with functional abdominal pain. Drossman (1996) recommended a treatment plan focused on the goal of gaining control over the symptoms rather than total cure. Encouragement of patient responsibility should be initiated via use of a behavioral diary measuring symptom severity and notation of degree of disability. A psychiatric consultation should be mandated before any surgical procedure is performed (Drossman 1996). Use of medications should be limited to antidepressants because analgesics and benzodiazepines are rarely effective, and both have abuse potential (Drossman 1996).

The couvade syndrome, found in men whose wives are pregnant, presents with acute gastrointestinal symptoms and may be mistaken for organic disease. The syndrome is characterized by nausea, vomiting, strange food cravings, abdominal bloating, and fatigue. In developing countries, couvade symptoms may be dramatic, with males taking to bed, but it may be far more subtle in developed countries. Risk factors for expectant fathers include low income, stress levels, poor health, ethnic minority status, and a greater number of children (Clinton 1986). Lipkin and Lamb (1982) showed that physicians often miss the relation of the symptoms to the patient's expectant fatherhood. Couvade is best managed by very conservative measures and reassurance that the gastrointestinal difficulties will remit following the birth of the child (Lipkin and Lamb 1982). Patients refractory to explanation and reassurance require psychiatric assessment and medical psychotherapy.

Functional dyspepsia is diagnosed when a patient complains of chronic upper abdominal pain, bloating, early satiety, fullness, or nausea. The Rome II (Table 2–3) classification requires persistent or recurrent pain or discomfort centered in the upper abdomen with no evidence of organic disease to explain the symptoms and no relief of the discomfort from defecation or changes in bowel movements. Selective hypersensitivity in the stomach but not duodenum may be a factor (Coffin et al. 1994).

Table 2–3.   Rome II criteria for functional dyspepsia

At least 12 weeks, which need not be consecutive, within the preceding 12 months of
1. Persistent or recurrent dyspepsia (pain or discomfort centered in the upper abdomen); and
2. No evidence of organic disease (including at upper endoscopy) that is likely to explain the symptoms; and
3. No evidence that dyspepsia is exclusively relieved by defecation or associated with onset of a change in stool frequency or stool form

Source.   Reprinted from Talley NJ, Stanghellini V, Heading RC, et al: "Functional Gastroduodenal Disorders." *Gut* 45(suppl II):II37–II42, 1999. Copyright 1999 by BMJ Publishing Group. Used with permission.

Psychological factors such as elevated levels of anxiety and depression as well as excessive internal monitoring of visceral sensations also partition functional dyspeptic patients from other populations (Herschbach et al. 1999). Depression and negative life events in such patients have been linked with abnormal vagal tone, which could be an etiological factor (Drossman 1982). Talley and colleagues (1986) carefully examined the association of such psychological factors in a group of patients with functional dyspepsia and a matched group with peptic ulcer disease. The functional dyspepsia patients had significantly more symptoms of anxiety and tension and higher scores for trait tension and hostility than did the peptic ulcer group.

No clearly established medical treatments are available for functional dyspepsia, but antacids, proton pump inhibitors, prokinetic agents, and eradication of *H. pylori* are used (McQuaid 1998). Patients with functional dyspepsia usually respond poorly to psychopharmacological agents other than antidepressants. It is particularly important to minimize the use of opiate medications. Supportive psychotherapy usually does not lead to persistent pain relief. Cognitive psychotherapy has been shown to improve both psychological and somatic distress in patients with this syndrome (Haug et al. 1994). Hamilton and colleagues (2000) reported that brief psychotherapy in which an interpersonal model is used significantly ameliorated both somatic and psychological symptoms. The only subgroup not to respond were those with severe heartburn.

Delayed gastric emptying may present with nausea, vomiting, bloating, postprandial fullness, early satiety, and anorexia. Etiologies include diabetic gastroparesis, gastroesophageal reflux, postvagotomy sequelae, and gastric ulcer. Depression may cause delayed gastric emptying, possibly because of increased vagal tone (Gorard et al. 1996). This abnormality also might explain why constipation is a common symptom of depression. Recent data suggest that women may be more prone to such delayed gut transit. Bennett et al. (2000) found that such patients had inhibited anger and elevated levels of depressed mood.

Patients with anorexia nervosa also have been shown to have delayed gastric emptying, possibly as a result of gastric neuromuscular involvement. Medications with significant anticholinergic activity, such as imipramine, may delay emptying. Treatment of delayed gastric emptying includes eliminating anticholinergic drugs and using promotility medications such as metoclopramide. Renutrition alone has been shown to improve gastric emptying in anorexia nervosa (Rigaud et al. 1988).

Food Allergies and Pseudo–Food Allergy

Many patients complain of gastrointestinal problems such as indigestion, nausea, and flatulence and attribute such symptoms to food allergies or malabsorptive syndromes resulting from enzyme deficiencies. Whether such beliefs are due to the phenomenon of foods fostering gut transit or true allergies is not known (Locke et al. 2000). Food allergies, which are more common in infants and children, are most often caused by eggs, cow's milk, legumes, and nuts. In adults, shellfish are reported to be common allergens. The evaluation for food allergy is subtle and requires carefully controlled challenges. Skin tests correlate poorly with the severity of symptomatology produced by foods.

Lactose intolerance is a common condition in which a variety of abdominal symptoms occur after ingestion of mammalian milk. Decreased lactase-phlorizin hydrolase (an enzyme that splits lactose into glucose and galactose) is the cause of this syndrome. The lactose absorption test is used to make the diagnosis. The lactose breath hydrogen test also elucidates lactose nonabsorption and is easier to carry out in children.

Treatment of food allergies consists of elimination of dietary allergens while maintaining a balanced diet. For lactose intolerance, use of enzyme substitutes such as yeast β-galactosidase can reduce symptoms when milk products are ingested. Several effective over-the-counter enzyme preparations are widely available.

In addition to the well-documented food allergies and lactose malabsorption syndromes, the syndrome of pseudo–food allergy has been described. Patients usually are women between ages 35 and 50 with a mild mood disorder. Rix et al. (1984) examined a series of patients complaining of food allergies and found that most did not have a definable allergy. Recently, Suarez and colleagues (1997) documented that patients claiming to be severely lactose intolerant often could tolerate one to two cups of milk per day.

Shorter (1997) reviewed the history of questionable beliefs of food allergies and believes that they were the precursor of the contemporary entity of multiple chemical sensitivity. Leznoff (1997) suggested that such putative allergies actually might be misattributed anxiety disorders. Meggs (1995), however, views such beliefs and reactions as a result of behavioral conditioning in the setting of depression. These patients are frequently somatizers. This false disease conviction can lead patients to seek out a variety of treatments that do not address the actual problem. Management includes paying careful attention to illness beliefs, treating any associated mood or anxiety symptoms, and ensuring a balanced diet because such patients often restrict their food intake to dangerously low nutritional levels.

A pernicious pseudo–food allergy by proxy has been described in which a parent falsely believes that a child is allergic to certain foods and allows only a diet that causes malnutrition. Gray and Bentovim (1996) reported on 41 children with various illness-induction syndromes, including one in which the parent makes an allegation of food allergy and as a result withholds food from the child.

Inflammatory Bowel Disease

Inflammatory bowel disease (IBD) encompasses regional enteritis (Crohn's disease) and ulcerative colitis. In Crohn's disease, the inflammation extends through the intestinal wall. It may affect any part of the gastrointestinal tract but most commonly involves the ileum and cecum. Principal symptoms of Crohn's disease include abdominal pain, diarrhea, and weight loss. The initial presentation may consist of months of an insidious course, including intermittent diarrhea and vague abdominal pain. There may be a significant discrepancy between subjective symptoms and objective signs of disease activity (e.g., endoscopic or radiographic studies) (Stenson 2000). Therefore, especially among patients with a personal or family history of the disease, it is important to treat for a suspected flare rather than attributing symptoms to somatization or an eating disorder.

Ulcerative colitis is confined to the mucosa and submucosa of the colon. The primary symptom of ulcerative colitis is diarrhea, which is usually accompanied by blood in the stool. The disease usually begins with nonbloody diarrhea progressing to bloody diarrhea. Like Crohn's disease, it is relapsing and remitting. Other symptoms include abdominal pain and fever. Colectomy cures the patient of the illness. The risk of colon cancer is much greater for patients with ulcerative colitis than for those with Crohn's disease, but both diseases carry a greater risk than the general population (Stenson 2000).

The peak age at onset for IBD is 15–25 years, with a second smaller peak between 55 and 65 years. The most important risk factor is a positive family history. Extraintestinal manifestations of IBD such as sclerosing cholangitis and ankylosing spondylitis may be quite debilitating (Stenson 2000).

For mild to moderate colonic or ileocolic Crohn's disease, medications may include sulfasalazine, mesalamine, azathioprine, and metronidazole. Prednisone may be given for nonresponders or those with severe disease (Stenson 2000). For ulcerative colitis, corticosteroids usually are used to treat active disease, and remission is maintained with sulfasalazine or related medications.

Psychiatric Factors

No well-controlled studies have found an association between ulcerative colitis and psychopathology (North et al. 1990). Nonetheless, stress may exacerbate symptoms for some patients. For example, Levenstein and colleagues (1994) found an association between rectal inflammation and perceived stress among patients with ulcerative colitis. Because this association was present even for asymptomatic patients, such a finding provides preliminary support for the view that life stress may cause verifiable tissue alterations in some patients.

Nutritional problems, treatment of chronic pain, and steroid treatment or withdrawal may cause or exacerbate psychiatric symptoms in these patients (see Table 2–1). Depression and fatigue often occur after the withdrawal of long-term steroid therapy (e.g., after successful colectomy). In such a case, the patient should first be evaluated for adrenal insufficiency. If this evaluation is negative, antidepressants should be considered. Ileal disease or resection of more than 100 cm of ileum may cause malabsorption, resulting in low serum vitamin B_{12} (Stenson 2000). This deficiency may be associated with psychiatric problems such as dementia.

The individual with Crohn's disease must cope with an uncertain and relentless disease that has exacerbations and remissions. The relatively favorable prognosis of the patient with ulcerative colitis after colectomy stands in contrast to that of the Crohn's disease patient, whose illness may persist. In one study, the three most prominent concerns of IBD patients were having an ostomy bag, a low energy level, and surgery (Drossman et al. 1989). Those with Crohn's disease were significantly more concerned with pain; patients with ulcerative colitis were significantly more concerned with loss of bowel control and developing cancer.

Use of intravenous hyperalimentation is sometimes necessary in fulminant cases of regional enteritis or for individuals with short bowel syndrome. Depression, fear, distortion of self-concept, loss of appetite, and marital stress are common in individuals who undergo total parenteral nutrition for periods of a few months or longer (Hall and Beresford 1987). Patients receiving chronic hyperalimentation also have been found to have mild cognitive impairment. These symptoms are due to metabolic problems, infection, or the disease that led to the need for total parenteral nutrition. Depression should be treated with antidepressants and psychotherapy. The presence of cognitive dysfunction should lead to a comprehensive assessment of fluid, electrolyte, and vitamin status, as well as screening for infection related to the central line.

In both ulcerative colitis and Crohn's disease, institution of an ostomy necessitates significant adaptation by the patient. Patients may react with shame, depression, and anger at the alteration of their excretory system. Before surgery, it is most helpful to have the ostomy therapist talk to both patient and spouse. Use of patient organizations, such as the United Ostomy Association or the Crohn's and Colitis Foundation of America, can be an invaluable adjunct to medical treatment. Such groups provide patient advocates who have had personal experience with their own ostomies and can aid the patient with concerns such as leakage, skin breakdown, and odors. Inclusion of the spouse is important in treating the patient with an ostomy. Studies have noted that men are more comfortable having their wives view their ostomy and appliance, whereas women seem to experience more shame (Schuster 1995).

Irritable Bowel Syndrome

IBS is diagnosed when an individual has abdominal pain that is relieved with defecation and is associated with a change in frequency or consistency of stool (see Rome II criteria in Table 2–4; cf. Drossman 1999). IBS, one of the functional bowel disorders (see Table 2–5), is diagnosed in more than 25% of ambulatory patients seen by gastroenterologists. In a national household survey, 7.7% of the men and 14.5% of the women met criteria for IBS (Drossman et al. 1993).

Table 2–4. Rome II criteria for irritable bowel syndrome

At least 12 weeks, which need not be consecutive, within the preceding 12 months of abdominal discomfort or pain that has two or three features:
1. Relieved with defecation; and/or
2. Onset associated with a change in the frequency of stool; and/or
3. Onset associated with a change in the form (appearance) of stool

Source.   Reprinted from Thompson WG, Longstreth GF, Drossman DA, et al: "Functional Bowel Disorders and Functional Abdominal Pain." *Gut* 45(suppl II):II43–II47, 1999. Copyright 1999 by BMJ Publishing Group. Used with permission.

IBS was classified as a functional bowel disorder because no clear evidence indicated that individuals with the syndrome have a primary disturbance of motility (Farthing 1995). Recent

Table 2–5. Rome II functional bowel disorders

Irritable bowel syndrome
Functional abdominal bloating
Functional constipation
Functional diarrhea
Unspecified functional bowel disorder

Source. Reprinted from Thompson WG, Longstreth GF, Drossman DA, et al: "Functional Bowel Disorders and Functional Abdominal Pain." *Gut* 45(suppl II):II43–II47, 1999. Copyright 1999 by BMJ Publishing Group. Used with permission.

fascinating research has shed light on the brain-gut interactions in the syndrome. Patients with IBS have been shown to have increased sensitivity to rectal distention (e.g., Whitehead et al. 1990). Functional magnetic resonance imaging studies have found that among patients with IBS, but not control subjects, painful rectal distention led to greater activation of the anterior cingulate cortex than did nonpainful stimuli (Mertz et al. 2000). The anterior cingulate cortex is a brain center involved with affective responses to pain. In other work, left prefrontal cortical activation occurred during anticipation of a noxious stimulus (Naliboff et al. 1998). In a series of studies, Blomhoff and colleagues (2000) assessed rectal wall reactivity and cortical evoked potentials to elucidate brain-gut interactions in IBS patients. IBS patients appear to have abnormal brain responses and rectal wall reactivity to emotional words. In addition, rectal wall reactivity is associated with frontal amplitude, supporting the notion that brain and gut interact intimately.

Although findings are not yet entirely consistent or definitive, studies such as these lend support to the notion that brain and gut are closely linked in IBS and that IBS patients centrally process rectal information differently from control subjects. It is possible that serotonin is a mediator of the brain-gut connection (cf. Kim and Camilleri 2000).

Many people who do not seek health care report bowel habits similar to those of patients with operationally defined IBS. Recent studies indicate that, whereas patients with IBS tend to have psychological problems, nonpatients who meet IBS criteria do not (Drossman et al. 1988; Farthing 1995; Herschbach et al. 1999). In a large study of patients with functional bowel disorders (most with IBS), Drossman et al. (2000) assessed factors associated with IBS severity. They found that more severe IBS was associated with extent of depression and the use of maladaptive coping strategies.

Noncolonic gastrointestinal symptoms such as nausea are often present in IBS, and extragastrointestinal symptoms are also common. IBS patients more commonly have other allied conditions associated with visceral hypersensitivity (e.g., fibromyalgia and interstitial cystitis); increased sensitivity in these conditions may be centrally mediated (Silverman et al. 1997). An alternative explanation is that patients with IBS overestimate their physical problems and seek medical care because of abnormal illness behavior rather than the disease itself. Patients with IBS have a marked tendency toward somatization (Lydiard et al. 1993). Rates of psychiatric disorder are higher than those seen among individuals with IBD (Walker et al. 1995). A recent study found that psychiatric illness was more common among relatives of patients with IBS than among those of a control group (Woodman et al. 1998). It appears that psychiatric illness often precedes the onset of gastrointestinal symptoms (Walker et al. 1990). Studies such as this one suggest that mental symptoms are associated with the disorder rather than merely a reaction to the discomfort of symptoms (for an excellent review, see Walker et al. 1990).

Sexual abuse histories are much more common in patients with IBS than in patients with IBD (Walker et al. 1993), and posttraumatic stress disorder is also frequently present in patients with IBS (Irwin et al. 1996). Child abuse is associated with the development of IBS in adults (Kendall-Tackett 2000). Physical, sexual, and emotional abuse in adulthood are associated with the presence of IBS (Ali et al. 2000). Gastrointestinal illness behavior also may be learned. In one recent study, children of parents with IBS had elevated levels of outpatient visits for abdominal pain and diarrhea (Levy et al. 2000)

Various treatments have been used for IBS. These include dietary management with high-fiber diets (to avoid gas-producing

legumes), bulking agents (e.g., Metamucil), anticholinergic anti-
spasmodics (e.g., hyoscyamine or dicyclomine), and loperamide.
Gastrointestinal symptoms in panic disorder patients, many of
which are consistent with IBS, have been shown to respond to antipanic pharmacotherapy (Noyes et al. 1990). Studies of psychotropics (e.g., TCAs) in IBS are generally not well designed, so it is
difficult to draw definitive conclusions about any particular
psychotropic agent (Jailwala et al. 2000). (See Table 2–6 for considerations in using psychotropics in various gastrointestinal diseases.) As noted earlier in this section, serotonin may be a
mediator of brain-gut interactions in IBS. Alosetron, a potent serotonin type 3 receptor antagonist, was recently shown to be
somewhat effective for this condition. Unfortunately, this medication was withdrawn from the market in 2000 because of multiple reports of ischemic colitis.

Table 2–6. Considerations in the use of psychotropic medications
among patients with gastrointestinal disease

Gastrointestinal condition	Implications for psychotropic use
Gastroesophageal reflux disease	Avoid medications with anticholinergic side effects
Delayed gastric emptying	Avoid medications with anticholinergic side effects
Irritable bowel syndrome— diarrhea predominant	Medications with anticholinergic side effects may be helpful
Irritable bowel syndrome— constipation predominant	Avoid medications with anticholinergic side effects
Chronic constipation	Avoid medications with anticholinergic side effects
Advanced liver disease	Use low doses of all medications metabolized by the liver; if benzodiazepines are needed, use those metabolized by conjugation (lorazepam, temazepam, oxazepam)
Hepatic encephalopathy	Avoid benzodiazepines

Irritable bowel complaints may respond to antidepressants regardless of whether the patient is clinically depressed. Medications with anticholinergic effects, such as imipramine, are preferred for diarrhea-predominant irritable bowel. Those with low anticholinergic effects, such as the selective serotonin reuptake inhibitors (SSRIs) (other than paroxetine) and bupropion, are preferred for patients with a constipation-predominant condition. Many patients who do not have concurrent major depression will respond symptomatically to relatively low doses of a cyclic antidepressant.

Cognitive-behavioral therapy (Payne and Blanchard 1995) and short-term dynamic psychotherapy (Guthrie et al. 1993) may be helpful for some patients. A combined approach that uses group therapy, relaxation therapy, and focal problem solving may diminish somatic concerns and anxiety in persons with IBS despite the persistence of symptoms (Wise et al. 1982). However, many studies that compare psychological treatment with a control group have methodological limitations (Talley et al. 1996). In patients with marked hypochondriacal concerns, prevention of excessive health-care seeking and scheduling of regular frequent primary care visits may be useful.

Hepatic Diseases

In this section, we focus on the neuropsychiatric manifestations of three liver disorders or syndromes: hepatic encephalopathy, alcoholic liver disease, and viral hepatic disease. In addition, we discuss the use of psychotropic medications in liver disease and the hepatotoxicity of various psychotropic agents.

Hepatic Encephalopathy

Hepatic encephalopathy is the major neuropsychiatric disorder that occurs in both acute and chronic liver failure. It is a form of delirium that occurs primarily in cirrhotic patients with portal hypertension and portosystemic shunting (Chung et al. 1995; Collis and Lloyd 1992; Gitlin 1996). The early stages of portosystemic encephalopathy are characterized by cognitive and attentional impairment with irritability and affective lability. Sleep disturbances, tremor, asterixis, and motor incoordination are also common in the early stages. Later stages are stupor and coma.

A subclinical hepatic encephalopathy also has been described. Subclinical hepatic encephalopathy cannot be detected through general clinical examination but requires specific neuropsychological and neurophysiological examination. Its prevalence among patients with cirrhosis is estimated to vary from 30% to 84%, depending on the methodology used to detect it. It is considered to be clinically relevant for two reasons. First, it could represent an early stage of clinical hepatic encephalopathy; and second, the psychomotor deficits found in subclinical hepatic encephalopathy could have a negative effect on patient's daily functioning. Patients with cirrhosis and subclinical hepatic encephalopathy reported significantly more impairment in all 12 scales of the Sickness Impact Profile (SIP) compared with cirrhotic patients without subclinical hepatic encephalopathy (Groeneweg et al. 1998). In this study, subclinical hepatic encephalopathy was defined by the presence of at least one abnormal psychometric test result and/or abnormal slowing of the electroencephalogram (EEG).

The laboratory screen for hepatic encephalopathy consists of liver function tests and serum ammonia levels. EEG may be helpful in questionable cases if it shows characteristic diffuse slowing and/or triphasic waves of metabolic delirium. However, these findings are not specific to hepatic encephalopathy (Gitlin 1996). Structural and functional neuroimaging techniques have been used in an effort to find early markers of brain damage in patients with subclinical hepatic encephalopathy. A recent study that used brain single photon emission computed tomography in cirrhotic patients with subclinical hepatic encephalopathy showed an increase in perfusion in some parts of the limbic system and in the brain regions with connections to the limbic system, such as the striatum and the mesial temporal regions, with neuropsychological impairment (Catafau et al. 2000).

Hepatic encephalopathy is generally thought to be multifactorial. Most theories about its etiology hypothesize that an alteration in the blood-brain barrier results in increased permeability to certain toxins (Chung et al. 1995; Collis and Lloyd 1992; Gitlin 1996). One theory proposes that several neurotoxins such as mercaptans, fatty acids, and ammonia act synergistically to produce encephalopathy. Although the mean arterial blood ammonia level is significantly increased in 90% of encephalopathic patients, it has been difficult to establish a close relation between the blood ammonia level and the severity of encephalopathy (Gitlin 1996). In addition, hepatic encephalopathy can be present in patients with a normal blood ammonia level. For these reasons, many clinicians rely more on clinical assessment to determine whether liver failure is the cause of delirium.

Another theory proposes that a deficit in neurotransmission is the cause. In acute liver failure, astrocytes undergo swelling, resulting in increased intracranial pressure, and the extracellular concentration of glutamate is increased. In chronic liver failure, the astrocyte undergoes characteristic changes known as Alzheimer type II astrocytosis. The astrocytes manifest altered expression of several proteins and enzymes, including monoamine oxidase B, glutamine synthetase, and peripheral-type benzodiazepine receptors. The expression of other neuroproteins, such as monoamine oxidase A and neuronal nitric oxide synthetase, is also modified. These changes have been attributed to the toxic effect of ammonia and manganese, the two substances that are normally removed by the hepatobiliary route. Manganese deposition in the globus pallidus in chronic liver failure results in signal hyperintensity on T1-weighted magnetic resonance imaging and may be responsible for extrapyramidal symptoms (Hazell and Butterworth 1999).

An additional theory proposes that false neurotransmitters (such as γ-aminobutyric acid [GABA], octopamine, serotonin, and histamine) displace dopamine and norepinephrine and alter brain function. In liver failure, the plasma concentrations of aromatic amino acids and tryptophan are increased relative to branched-chain amino acids. Because aromatic and branched-chain amino acids compete for the same carrier across the blood-brain barrier, a relative increase in aromatic amino acids occurs in the brain. The increased phenylalanine (an aromatic amino acid) inhibits tyrosine 3-hydroxylase, the rate-limiting step in the synthesis of catecholamines. Tyrosine begins to accumulate and is then metabolized by alternative pathways into the false neurotransmitters. Based on this theory, infusion of branched-chain amino acids has been tried, with mixed results, for treatment of hepatic encephalopathy (Chung et al. 1995; Gitlin 1996).

The benzodiazepine hypothesis postulates that the liver's inability to metabolize endogenous benzodiazepines results in increased levels of circulating benzodiazepines. Based on this hypothesis, flumazenil, a GABA antagonist, has been used, with mixed results, to treat hepatic encephalopathy (see, e.g., Gyr et al. 1996; Van der Rijt et al. 1995). Because only a subgroup will respond, flumazenil cannot serve as a diagnostic probe. Because it is expensive and would need to be given continuously by intravenous infusion, it also cannot be used for ongoing therapy. Finally, in recent research that used proton magnetic resonance spectroscopy, clinically diagnosed hepatic encephalopathy correlated with low levels of choline and *myo*-inositol in the brain (Ross et al. 1996).

Numerous factors and conditions can precipitate acute hepatic encephalopathy: gastrointestinal bleed, dehydration, dietary protein overload, infection, electrolyte abnormalities, and benzodiazepines. Treatment of hepatic encephalopathy involves both direct and supportive measures. The main aim is to reduce the ammonia load with treatments such as a low-protein diet and lactulose. Antibiotics may be used to clear the colon of bacteria in an effort to decrease the ammonia load. For agitation, low-dose, high-potency antipsychotics such as haloperidol are recommended. The efficacy and safety of the newer atypical antipsychotic medications in these patients have not yet been studied. Benzodiazepines may worsen the encephalopathy. The risk is greatest with those benzodiazepines metabolized primarily by oxidation, given the impaired liver function in these patients.

Alcoholic Liver Disease

Alcohol abuse is the most common cause of liver disease in Western societies. About 18 million Americans abuse alcohol. Among alcoholic persons, 75% of all medical deaths result from liver cirrhosis. Alcoholic liver disease peaks between ages 40 and 55, with a male-to-female ratio of 3:1 (Crabb and Lumeng 1995).

Alcoholic liver disease can be divided into three stages, which are defined histologically: fatty liver, hepatitis, and cirrhosis. Alcoholic fatty liver is generally a benign reversible form of liver disease characterized by the accumulation of large droplets of fat in the hepatocytes. It is found in 75% of alcoholic patients and presents clinically with hepatomegaly (Crabb and Lumeng 1995).

Alcoholic hepatitis is the second stage of alcoholic liver disease and is more serious. Histologically, it involves ballooning degeneration and necrosis of the hepatocytes. Patients generally present clinically with anorexia, malaise, weakness, nausea, jaundice, abdominal pain, weight loss, and fever. Others may present with hepatic failure, bleeding esophageal varices, hepatic encephalopathy, and ascites, which lead to rapid death (Crabb and Lumeng 1995). Treatment of the acute episodes involves supportive measures, as well as administration of amino acids, corticosteroids, anabolic steroids, and propylthiouracil. Abstinence from alcohol is essential for long-term treatment (Crabb and Lumeng 1995).

The third stage of alcoholic liver disease is alcoholic cirrhosis, characterized by fibrosis throughout the liver. For a period of time, patients may be asymptomatic, but 10%–20% of patients have complications and stigmata of liver disease (Crabb and Lumeng 1995). Prognosis depends largely on abstinence from alcohol and the presence of jaundice, ascites, and gastrointestinal bleeding, which are predictors of 5-year survival. A formal family intervention should be considered.

The definitive treatment for end-stage alcoholic liver disease (hepatic cirrhosis) is liver transplantation. It necessitates comprehensive evaluation, including psychiatric evaluation, of potential liver transplantation recipients and donors and discussion of the risks and benefits of the procedure, prognosis, life after transplantation, and psychosocial issues related to liver transplantation. Most centers will perform liver transplantations on candidates with 6 months (or even less) of sobriety, insight into alcohol drinking as a problem, maintenance and monitoring of sobriety, and strong social support for remaining sober. (Extensive discussion of psychiatric aspects of liver transplantation is beyond the scope of this chapter.)

Viral Hepatic Disease

Viral infections, such as hepatitis B and C viruses, can cause serious hepatic disease. Hepatitis C virus (HCV) infection is the most common cause of chronic liver disease in the United States. An estimated 1.8% of the United States population carries the antibody for HCV, and more than 70% of those remain chronically infected (Sarbah and Younossi 2000). Twenty-five percent of HCV-infected individuals progress to cirrhosis, with an estimated 8,000–10,000 deaths every year. Injection drug use is the most common route of transmission and currently accounts for most of the new cases. HCV infection is found in more than 50% of injection drug users (National Institutes of Health 1997).

Most acute infections with hepatitis C and B viruses are asymptomatic despite elevations in liver enzyme levels. Of those with newly acquired HCV infection, 30% develop symptoms such as malaise, loss of appetite, and jaundice. Acute hepatitis C rarely causes fulminant liver failure. The acute episode resolves in 15% of patients, and the rest develop chronic hepatitis. In chronic hepatitis C, 20% of infected patients have clinical liver disease, 50% are asymptomatic but have increased liver enzyme levels, and 30% are asymptomatic and have normal liver enzyme levels (National Institutes of Health 1997). The progression of chronic hepatitis C is slow; some patients may have no clinical indication of infection until they develop cirrhosis-related complications such as hepatic encephalopathy, jaundice, and ascites. It is currently the leading cause of chronic liver disease in the United States and the most common indication for liver transplantation.

Clinically significant depression has been reported in patients with hepatitis C who have end-stage liver disease. In their retrospective review, D.H. Lee et al. (1997) reported that 24% of 359 untreated HCV-infected patients were depressed, and two-thirds required antidepressant treatment. In a recent prospective study of 82 liver transplant candidates, Singh et al. (1997) found that patients with HCV were significantly younger, had greater somatic manifestations of the illness (e.g., pain), and had higher levels of depressive symptoms compared with those with end-stage liver disease from other causes. In addition, depression has been found to be more common among patients with recurrent HCV after liver transplantation than in those without the virus (Singh et al. 1999).

Patients with some psychiatric disorders appear to have a higher prevalence of HCV infection than do patients without psychiatric disorders. In a large retrospective study, 6.7% of the patients hospitalized for mental retardation, psychosis, and dementia were infected with HCV. Among these diagnoses, psychosis was the most important independent risk factor for HCV infection (Cividini et al. 1997). Heavy alcohol drinking has been shown to worsen hepatic injury and may accelerate progression of HCV infection (Schiff 1997).

The standard treatment for chronic hepatitis B and C is interferon alpha (with or without ribavirin). Treatment is aimed at reducing inflammation and liver cell damage, thus preventing cirrhosis and hepatocellular carcinoma. However, interferon alpha alone produces a response in only 40% of the patients with hepatitis C. Furthermore, more than 90% of the patients relapse soon after stopping therapy. The synthetic nucleoside analogue ribavirin has been used in combination with interferon alpha; outcomes improved in both initial treatment and retreatment after relapse following monotherapy (Dieperink et al. 2000).

Estimates of the incidence of neuropsychiatric side effects in patients treated with interferon alpha range from 0% to 70%. These side effects include cognitive impairment, anxiety, depression, irritability, and mood lability (Trask et al. 2000). These neuropsychiatric sequelae are common reasons for discontinuation of interferon alpha therapy. Less commonly, patients receiving interferon alpha develop severe neuropsychiatric side effects, including confusion, lethargy, impaired mental state, severe depression, mania, and, on occasion, suicidality, especially with repeated administration of high doses (Trask et al. 2000). Completed and attempted suicides have been reported in several cases (e.g., Bourat et al. 1995; Janssen et al. 1994). There is controversy as to whether a history of psychiatric illness is a risk factor for development of neuropsychiatric sequelae with interferon alpha treatment (Valentine et al. 1998; see Table 2–1).

The specific mechanisms responsible for the beneficial effects and, in contrast, the development of neuropsychiatric side effects of interferon alpha are unknown. Because interferon alpha does not cross the blood-brain barrier, direct action of this agent on the brain cannot be responsible for the neuropsychiatric side effects. Several interesting theories have been proposed to explain these neuropsychiatric side effects: opioid-dopamine changes, serotonin depletion, norepinephrine increases, and endocrine dysfunction involving thyroid hormones, corticotropin, and cortisol (Trask et al. 2000).

The development of serious neuropsychiatric symptoms often requires discontinuation of the interferon alpha. In most cases, these symptoms abate within 2–3 weeks of discontinuation of interferon alpha (Trask et al. 2000). Identifying the neuropsychiatric symptoms early increases the opportunity to treat the side effects and help patients complete interferon alpha therapy. First, the clinician should attempt to reduce the dose of interferon alpha before discontinuing the medication completely, especially with mild neuropsychiatric side effects. However, depression should be treated aggressively with antidepressants concurrently with reducing the dose of interferon alpha (Lerner et al. 1999). Although no placebo-controlled studies of the use of antidepressants for treatment of interferon alpha–induced depression have been done, there have been several case reports of successful treatment of depression with TCAs and SSRIs in patients receiving interferon alpha for HCV infection. In addition, there have been reports on the use of methylphenidate for irritability and of antipsychotics for delirium, paranoia, and agitation (Fattovich et al. 1996; Valentine et al. 1998).

Many patients with chronic hepatitis B or C virus, whether or not they are symptomatic, experience some psychological distress. The presence of the infection may be perceived as affecting the individual's social status, leading to social isolation. The psychological difficulties include fatigue, depression, and demoralization, combined with difficulties in sexual functioning because of the fear of transmitting infection (Collis and Lloyd 1992). All patients with hepatitis B or C warrant testing for human immunodeficiency virus because the two diseases are transmitted by the same routes and are prevalent in the same population.

Psychotropic Medications in Patients With Liver Disease

The effect of hepatic insufficiency on the metabolism of psychotropic agents depends primarily on two factors: 1) the relative importance of the liver compared with the kidney in the drug metabolism and 2) the type of biotransformation a drug undergoes in the liver. Except for lithium salts, all psychotropic medications are metabolized primarily by the liver (Shen 1997); therefore, hepatic insufficiency may affect their metabolism. More recently, gabapentin (a new antiepileptic medication approved for use as an adjuvant treatment for complex partial seizures) has been used for psychiatric conditions, including anxiety disorders and bipolar illness. This medication is primarily metabolized and excreted by the kidneys; therefore, hepatic insufficiency does not affect its metabolism.

In liver disease, the reasons for change in pharmacokinetics are 1) changes in liver blood flow, 2) changes in quantity and affinity of binding proteins, 3) changes in volume of distribution with formation of peritoneal ascites (Beliles and Stoudemire 1998; Stoudemire and Moran 1998), and 4) changes in hepatic biotransformation of the psychotropic agents. Two main processes are involved in biotransformation: 1) enzymatic oxidation and 2) conjugation with an endogenous substrate such as glucuronic acid (Schwartz et al. 1997). Although hepatic enzymes involved in conjugation are well preserved, even in the presence of liver disease, hepatic enzymes that are involved in oxidation (i.e., the cytochrome P450 systems) are affected by different liver diseases and definitely by liver failure (Schwartz et al. 1997). Because conjugation is preserved in hepatic insufficiency, psychotropic medications that are primarily metabolized by glucuronidation can be used safely and with little dose adjustment.

The only psychotropic agents metabolized solely by conjugation are the benzodiazepines lorazepam, temazepam, and oxazepam (Crabb and Lumeng 1995; Schwartz et al. 1997).

Oxidation is the main metabolic transformation for all other psychotropic agents that are metabolized by the liver (Shen 1997). Therefore, the effects of hepatic insufficiency on peak levels, drug half-life, metabolically mediated drug activation and deactivation, and metabolite accumulation must be considered (Shen 1997). Most psychotropic medications are deactivated by hepatic oxidation, but some agents (e.g., amitriptyline and imipramine) undergo biotransformation to form active metabolites (Schwartz et al. 1997).

Even with relatively safe psychotropic medications such as SSRIs, it is advisable to use lower doses in patients with liver disease and hepatic insufficiency because, in these patients, the medications have been found to have increased plasma levels and longer half-lives (Chung et al. 1995). It has generally been recommended that TCAs be used at reduced doses (Crabb and Lumeng 1995). Benzodiazepines, other than those metabolized solely by conjugation, should be used at reduced doses in hepatic insufficiency given that their clearance may be reduced by one-third to two-thirds (Crabb and Lumeng 1995; Schwartz et al. 1997).

Although alterations in biotransformation of psychotropic agents are the main determinants of altered pharmacokinetics in hepatic insufficiency, drug elimination also depends on delivery of drugs to the liver. Patients with hepatic insufficiency have portosystemic shunting with loss of first-pass metabolism, which makes many drugs reach systemic circulation at higher concentrations than they normally would when taken orally (Schwartz et al. 1997). This particularly affects psychotropic medications that are very efficiently extracted by the liver (e.g., TCAs) compared with agents that are poorly extracted (e.g., benzodiazepines).

In general, given the altered pharmacokinetics and biotransformation of most psychotropic medications in hepatic insufficiency, these agents should be used cautiously. The clinician should use lower than normal initial dosages, wait longer than normal intervals before increasing dosages, and check blood levels frequently if they are available for the psychotropic drugs in question. Whenever possible, he or she also should use psychotropic agents that would not be significantly affected by hepatic disease.

Hepatotoxicity of Psychotropic Medications

Drugs with the potential for producing hepatotoxicity may be divided, in general, into two groups: direct hepatotoxins and indirect hepatotoxins (Beliles and Stoudemire 1998; Stoudemire and Moran 1998). Direct hepatotoxins produce liver damage and necrosis of a particular region of the liver in a dose-dependent fashion. Idiosyncratic or indirect hepatotoxins produce liver injury even when administered within the therapeutic range; the liver damage is generally diffuse and associated with inflammation. Hepatotoxicity is caused by the accumulation of a toxic metabolite (Bass and Ockner 1996).

Hepatotoxicity of psychotropic drugs occurs in a variable, but small, proportion of users and is unpredictable or idiosyncratic. When hepatotoxicity occurs in association with rash, eosinophilia, or a rapid positive rechallenge, sufficient evidence exists to ascribe the mechanism to an immune-mediated hypersensitivity reaction. Hepatotoxicity of psychotropic medications usually takes the form of hepatitis (destruction of liver parenchyma), cholestasis (impaired bile secretion), or both. Certain psychotropic drugs have the characteristic patterns of hepatitis (e.g., clozapine and tacrine), cholestasis (e.g., chlorpromazine, haloperidol, and TCAs), or a combined picture of hepatitis and cholestasis (e.g., diazepam) (Selim and Kaplowitz 1999). Hepatotoxicity of psychotropic medications may range from mild asymptomatic elevation of liver transaminases to fulminant hepatic necrosis, with hepatic encephalopathy and liver failure leading to death or requiring liver transplantation (Mayoral and Lewis 2000; Selim and Kaplowitz 1999).

Some antidepressant medications have been found to be hepatotoxic. The monoamine oxidase inhibitor tranylcypromine has been reported to cause hepatitis (Bass and Ockner 1996).

Most TCAs are potentially hepatotoxic. Imipramine can induce cholestatic jaundice that is generally not progressive (Selim and Kaplowitz 1999). Asymptomatic subclinical elevations of the transaminases occur in approximately 10% of the patients taking any TCA and in 25% of the patients taking imipramine, and cross-sensitization among TCAs may occur (Bass and Ockner 1996). Trazodone also has been implicated in mostly reversible liver injury with a pattern of both hepatitis and cholestasis (Bass and Ockner 1996; Selim and Kaplowitz 1999). Hepatotoxicity from SSRIs is very rare. With the newer generation antidepressants, there have been fewer case reports. Nefazodone also has been implicated in causing severe hepatotoxicity, with liver failure requiring liver transplantation and even leading to death in some case reports (e.g., Aranda-Michel et al. 1999). Because of multiple case reports of pemoline, a psychostimulant, causing hepatotoxicity, the level of serum aminotransferases should be monitored throughout the treatment with this agent (Bass and Ockner 1996).

For many years, it has been known that chlorpromazine may cause hepatic damage. Benign transaminase elevations may occur in up to 50% of those who take chlorpromazine chronically. The incidence of chlorpromazine-induced cholestatic jaundice ranges from 0.5% to 2%. The jaundice usually begins 2–5 weeks after the treatment has begun. This jaundice is almost always rapidly reversible on discontinuation of the medication. Chronic jaundice may occur but usually resolves within a few years (Bass and Ockner 1996). Other phenothiazines may cause hepatotoxicity, but they do so at a lower rate than does chlorpromazine (Jones et al. 1983). Hepatic dysfunction due to nonphenothiazine antipsychotics is rare (Bass and Ockner 1996). Of the newer atypical antipsychotics, clozapine has been reported to increase alanine aminotransferase in a mild and transient way in up to 37% of patients (Hummer et al. 1997). This appears to be benign, but toxic hepatitis also has been described (Panagiotis 1999). Case reports of risperidone-induced hepatotoxicity have ranged from mild elevation of liver transaminases to severe hepatotoxicity (e.g., Geller and Zuiderwijk 1998; Szigethy et al. 1999).

Tacrine, a reversible acetylcholinesterase inhibitor used in

Alzheimer's disease, has been associated with reversible increases in transaminases in up to 50% of patients within 7–12 weeks of beginning treatment. These laboratory abnormalities are generally asymptomatic and are rarely associated with jaundice. Most individuals who experience these liver enzyme elevations have been able to restart treatment successfully after the enzymes normalize (Bass and Ockner 1996). There are specific recommendations regarding obtaining baseline liver function tests prior to using this medication and checking liver functions during treatment. Because of its hepatotoxicity, tacrine is no longer a preferred treatment for Alzheimer's disease.

Carbamazepine has been found to cause mild asymptomatic elevations of liver transaminases in 5%–10% of patients (Stoudemire et al. 1991). The antiepileptic drug hypersensitivity syndrome has been described in patients receiving carbamazepine and phenytoin. The incidence is approximately 1 in 3,000 individuals. It is defined by the presence of fever, skin rash, and internal organ involvement, including the liver, in 35%–95% of cases. The clinical course is variable, but toxicity has been described, including fatal hepatic injury. When hepatitis is part of the syndrome, mortality rates have been as high as 20% (Mayoral and Lewis 2000). It is essential to obtain baseline liver function tests before using carbamazepine and regularly thereafter, more frequently early in the treatment. For a patient with underlying liver disease, carbamazepine would be relatively contraindicated. Because of the multiple potential drug-drug interactions with carbamazepine, it should be used cautiously with other medications with hepatotoxic effects.

Valproate causes transient, mild, asymptomatic transaminase elevations in approximately 10% of patients. This usually occurs after 10–12 weeks of therapy, and it is dose-dependent in some cases. Spontaneous recovery almost always occurs, and fatalities are rare. There have been cases of hepatic failure resulting from the use of valproate, but these have generally been in children younger than 2 years taking multiple anticonvulsants. Routine monitoring of liver tests is advisable, especially during the first 6 months of therapy (Bass and Ockner 1996).

Lamotrigine, one of the newer antiepileptic medications, has been used as a mood stabilizer in bipolar disorder and depression. A few case reports of reversible hepatotoxicity have been reported in adults and children during treatment with this medication, with or without associated multisystem failure and central nervous system conditions (Fayad et al. 2000).

Carcinoma of the Pancreas

Carcinoma of the pancreas is a particularly deadly disease. The incidence of pancreatic cancer is between 11 and 12 per 100,000 persons (DiMagno 1996). The national 5-year survival has increased from 1% to 3% in whites and from 3% to 5% in blacks in the past decade. Carcinoma of the pancreas is the fourth and the fifth most common cancer in men and in women, respectively, and has the lowest 5-year survival rate of any cancer. The incidence is increasing in women but has stabilized in men (American Gastroenterological Association 1999). It occurs more frequently in men than in women (1.5:1). The dismal survival of patients with pancreatic cancer is caused by late diagnosis and low resection rates (American Gastroenterological Association 1999). Approximately 80% of the cases of pancreatic cancer occur between ages 60 and 80, and cases in those younger than 40 are rare.

Risk factors for pancreatic cancer include idiopathic and alcoholic chronic pancreatitis, new-onset diabetes mellitus (less than 2 years, no family history, age>50 years), cigarette smoking, family history of nonpolyposis colon cancer, and hereditary pancreatitis in patients who are older than 45 years with paternal inheritance (American Gastroenterological Association 1999; DiMagno 1996). The suspicion of pancreatic cancer arises because of symptoms of pain, jaundice, anorexia with unexplained weight loss, depression, and anxiety. Screening blood work includes liver function tests and pancreatic enzymes. The tumor marker CA 19-9 has the greatest sensitivity (70%) and specificity (87%) for diagnosis of pancreatic cancer. Definitive diagnosis is usually made by dual-phase spiral computed tomography scan of the abdomen (sensitivity around 90%), and the most accurate imaging test for diagnosis is endoscopic ultrasonography, which has sensitivity and specificity of 99% and 100%, respectively (American Gastroenterological Association 1999).

Depressed mood and anxiety symptoms are believed to occur more commonly in patients with pancreatic cancer than in patients with other cancers. In assessing the prevalence of psychological distress by cancer site, Zabora et al. (2001) used the Brief Symptom Inventory as a component of comprehensive cancer care in 4,496 patients with cancer, comparing psychological distress among 14 cancer diagnoses. They found that pancreatic cancer patients produced the highest mean scores for depressive and anxiety symptoms. The prevalence of mood symptoms in pancreatic cancer patients generally has been around 50% (e.g., Joffee et al. 1986; Kelsen et al. 1995). In comparison, the prevalence of depression associated with cancer at other sites ranged from 1% in acute leukemia to 40% in oropharyngeal cancer (McDaniel et al. 1995). Pain, which is found in 80% of the patients with pancreatic cancer, has been found to correlate significantly with depression (Kelsen et al. 1995).

In their seminal review of the literature, Green and Austin (1993) found that in addition to the high prevalence of depression and anxiety among patients with pancreatic cancer, 33% presented with psychiatric symptoms before their initial physical complaints, and 43% presented with psychiatric and somatic symptoms concomitantly. Passik and Roth (1999) reported the first case of panic attacks developing in a patient with no psychiatric history just before the diagnosis of pancreatic cancer.

There has been much speculation about the existence of a link between physiological dysfunction of the pancreas and the generation of depressive and anxious states. Mood changes have been noted in patients who did not have knowledge of their diagnosis, suggesting that existential factors do not entirely explain the development of psychological disturbances in these patients. Some authors have suggested that a paraneoplastic syndrome might account for altered mood states (Petty and Noyes 1981). Others have suggested that the underlying mechanism could be autoimmune. According to this hypothesis, antibodies produced against a protein released by pancreatic cancer cells possess cross-reactivity with central nervous system tissues such as serotonin receptors, thereby altering mood states (Brown and Paraskevas 1982). Other theories implicate systemic bicarbonate shunting in the case of anxiety symptoms and hormonal and neurotransmitter abnormalities that involve corticotropin, parathyroid hormone, thyroid-releasing hormones, glucagon, serotonin, and insulin in the case of depression (Green and Austin 1993; Passik and Breitbart 1996).

The treatment implications of these possible psychobiological causes of depression and anxiety in pancreatic cancer are not entirely clear. There have been no placebo-controlled trials of the use of antidepressants in this population. There is no specific indication for one class of antidepressants over another, but the possibility of a serotonin-based mechanism causing mood and anxiety symptoms in this patient population suggests that SSRIs might have a theoretical advantage (Passik and Roth 1999). The choice of an antidepressant, for now, must continue to be based more on specific aspects of the patient's clinical presentation, the target symptoms, and avoidance of certain drug side effects. Further research in this area may help shed light on basic mechanisms of depression and anxiety in pancreatic cancer patients, as well as possible treatments.

References

Ali A, Toner BB, Stuckless N, et al: Emotional abuse, self-blame, and self-silencing in women with irritable bowel syndrome. Psychosom Med 62:76–82, 2000

American Gastroenterological Association: American Gastroenterological Association medical position statement: epidemiology, diagnosis, and treatment of pancreatic ductal adenocarcinoma. Gastroenterology 117:1463–1484, 1999

Aranda-Michel J, Koehler A, Bejarano B, et al: Nefazodone-induced liver failure: report of three cases. Ann Intern Med 130:285–288, 1999

Bass NM, Ockner RK: Drug-induced liver disease, in Hepatology: A Textbook of Liver Disease, Vol I, 3rd Edition. Edited by Zakim D, Boyer TD. Philadelphia, PA, WB Saunders, 1996, pp 962–1017

Bassotti G, Whitehead WE: Biofeedback as a treatment approach to gastrointestinal tract disorders. Am J Gastroenterol 89:158–164, 1994

Beliles KE, Stoudemire A: Psychopharmacologic treatment of depression in the medically ill. Psychosomatics 39:S2–19, 1998

Bennett EJ, Evans P, Scott AM, et al: Psychological and sex features of delayed gut transit in functional gastrointestinal disorders. Gut 46:83–87, 2000

Blomhoff S, Spetalen S, Jacobsen M, et al: Rectal tone and brain information processing in irritable bowel syndrome. Dig Dis Sci 45:1153–1159, 2000

Bourat L, Larrey D, Michel H: Attempted suicide during treatment of chronic viral hepatitis C with interferon (letter). Gastroenterol Clin Biol 19:1063, 1995

Brown JH, Paraskevas F: Cancer and depression: cancer presenting with depressive illness: an autoimmune disease? Br J Psychiatry 141:227–232, 1982

Cannon RO, Quyyumi AA, Mincemoyer R, et al: Imipramine in patients with chest pain despite normal coronary angiograms. N Engl J Med 330:1411–1417, 1994

Catafau AM, Kulisevsky J, Berna L, et al: Relationship between cerebral perfusion in frontal-limbic-basal ganglia circuits and neuropsychologic impairment in patients with subclinical hepatic encephalopathy. J Nucl Med 41:405–410, 2000

Chung RT, Jaffe DL, Friedman LS: Complications of chronic liver disease. Crit Care Clin 11:431–463, 1995

Cividini A, Pistorio A, Regazzetti A, et al: Hepatitis C virus infection among institutionalized psychiatric patients: a regression analysis of indicators of risk. J Hepatol 27:455–463, 1997

Clinton JF: Expectant fathers at risk for couvade. Nurs Res 35: 290–295, 1986

Clouse RE, Richter JE, Heading RC, et al: Functional esophageal disorders. Gut 45 (suppl 2):31–36, 1999

Coffin B, Azpiroz F, Guarner F, et al: Selective gastric hypersensitivity and reflex hyporeactivity in functional dyspepsia. Gastroenterology 107:1345–1351, 1994

Cohen S, Parkman HP: Diseases of the esophagus, in Cecil Textbook of Medicine, 21st Edition. Edited by Goldman L, Bennett, JC. Philadelphia, PA, WB Saunders, 2000, pp 658–667

Collis I, Lloyd G: Psychiatric aspects of liver disease. Br J Psychiatry 161:12–22, 1992

Crabb DW, Lumeng L: Alcoholic liver disease, in Bockus Gastroenterology, 5th Edition, Vol 3. Edited by Haubrich WS, Schaffner F, Berk JE. Philadelphia, PA, WB Saunders, 1995, pp 2215–2245

Dieperink E, Willenbring M, Ho SB: Neuropsychiatric symptoms associated with hepatitis C and interferon alfa: a review. Am J Psychiatry 157:867–876, 2000

DiMagno EB: Carcinoma of the pancreas, in Cecil Textbook of Medicine, 20th Edition, Vol 2. Edited by Bennett JC, Plum F. Philadelphia, Saunders, 1996, Chap 108

Drossman DA: Patients with psychogenic abdominal pain: six years observation in the medical setting. Am J Psychiatry 139:1549–1557, 1982

Drossman DA: Chronic functional abdominal pain. Am J Gastroenterol 91:2270–2271, 1996

Drossman DA: Do psychosocial factors define symptom severity and patient status in irritable bowel syndrome? Am J Med 107(5A):41S–50S, 1999

Drossman DA, McKee DC, Sandler RS, et al: Psychosocial factors in the irritable bowel syndrome. Gastroenterology 95:701–708, 1988

Drossman DA, Patrick DL, Mitchell CM, et al: Health-related quality of life in inflammatory bowel disease. Dig Dis Sci 34:1379–1386, 1989

Drossman DA, Lesserman J, Nachman G, et al: Sexual and physical abuse in women with functional or organic gastrointestinal disorders. Ann Intern Med 113:828–833, 1990

Drossman DA, Li Z, Andruzzi E, et al: U.S. householder survey of functional gastrointestinal disorders. Dig Dis Sci 38:1569–1580, 1993

Drossman DA, Creed FH, Olden KW, et al: Psychosocial aspects of the functional gastrointestinal disorders. Gut 45 (suppl II):1121–1130, 1999

Drossman DA, Lesserman J, Zhiming L, et al: Effects on coping on health outcome among women with gastrointestinal disorders. Psychosom Med 62:309–317, 2000

Farthing JG: Irritable bowel, irritable body, or irritable brain? BMJ 310:171–175, 1995

Fattovich G, Giustina G, Favarato S, et al: A survey of adverse events in 11,241 patients with chronic viral hepatitis treated with alfa interferon. J Hepatol 24:38–47, 1996

Fayad M, Choueiri R, Mikati M: Potential hepatotoxicity of lamotrigine. Pediatr Neurol 22:49–52, 2000

Fonagu P, Calloway SP: The effect of emotional arousal on spontaneous swallowing rates. J Psychosom Res 30:183–188, 1986

Geller WK, Zuiderwijk PB: Risperidone-induced hepatotoxicity. J Am Acad Child Adolesc Psychiatry 37:246–247, 1998, pp 605–617

Gorard DA, Gomborone JE, Libby GW, et al: Intestinal transit in anxiety and depression. Gut 39:551–555, 1996

Gray J, Bentovim A: Illness induction syndrome: paper I—a series of 41 children from 37 families identified at The Great Ormond Street Hospital for Children NHS Trust. Child Abuse Negl 20:655–673, 1996

Green AI, Austin CP: Psychopathology of pancreatic cancer: a psychobiologic probe. Psychosomatics 34:208–221, 1993

Groeneweg M, Quero JC, De Bruijn I, et al: Subclinical hepatic encephalopathy impairs daily functioning. Hepatology 28:45–49, 1998

Guthrie E, Creed F, Dawson D, et al: A randomised controlled trial of psychotherapy in patients with refractory irritable bowel syndrome. Br J Psychiatry 163:315–321, 1993

Gyr K, Meier R, Haussler J, et al: Evaluation of the efficacy and safety of flumazenil in the treatment of portal systemic encephalopathy: a double-blind, randomized, placebo controlled multicentre study. Gut 39:319–324, 1996

Hall RCW, Beresford TP: Psychiatric factors in the management of long-term hyperalimentation patients. Psychiatry in Medicine 5:211–217, 1987

Hamilton J, Guthrie E, Creed F, et al: A randomized controlled trial of psychotherapy in patients with functional dyspepsia. Gastroenterology 119:661–669, 2000

Haug TT, Wilhelmsen I, Svebak S, et al: Psychotherapy in functional dyspepsia. J Psychosom Res 38:735–744, 1994

Hazell AS, Butterworth RF: Hepatic encephalopathy: an update of pathophysiologic mechanisms. Proc Soc Exp Biol Med 222:99–112, 1999

Herschbach P, Henrich G, vonRad M: Psychological factors in functional gastrointestinal disorders: characteristics of the disorder or of the illness behavior? Psychosom Med 61:148–153, 1999

Hummer M, Kury M, Kurzthaler I, et al: Hepatotoxicity of clozapine. J Clin Psychopharmacol 17:314–317, 1997

Irwin C, Falsetti SA, Lydiard RB, et al: Comorbidity of posttraumatic stress disorder and irritable bowel syndrome. J Clin Psychiatry 57:576–578, 1996

Jailwala J, Imperiale T, Kroenke K: Pharmacologic treatment of the irritable bowel syndrome: a systematic review of randomized, controlled trials. Ann Intern Med 133:136–147, 2000

Janssen HL, Brouwer JT, Van Der Mast RC, et al: Suicide associated with alpha-interferon therapy for chronic viral hepatitis. J Hepatol 21:241–243, 1994

Jenkins PLG: Psychogenic abdominal pain. Gen Hosp Psychiatry 13:27–30, 1991

Joffee RT, Rubinow DR, Denicoff KD, et al: Depression and carcinoma of the pancreas. Gen Hosp Psychiatry 8:241–245, 1986

Jones JK, Van de Carr SW, Zimmerman M, et al: Hepatotoxicity associated with phenothiazines. Psychopharmacol Bull 19:24–27, 1983

Kahrilas P: Gastroesophageal reflux disease and its complications, in Sleisenger and Fordtran's Gastrointestinal and Liver Disease, 6th Edition. Edited by Feldman M, Scharschmidt BF, Sleisenger MH, et al. Philadelphia, PA, WB Saunders, 1998, pp 498–514

Katz PO: Disorders of the esophagus: dysphagia, noncardiac chest pain, and gastroesophageal reflux, in Principles of Ambulatory Medicine, 4th Edition. Edited by Barker LR, Burton JR, Zieve PD. Baltimore, MD, Williams & Wilkins, 1995a, pp 435–446

Katz PO: Peptic ulcer disease, in Principles of Ambulatory Medicine, 4th Edition. Edited by Barker LR, Burton JR, Zieve PD. Baltimore, MD, Williams & Wilkins, 1995b, pp 456–458

Kelsen DP, Portenoy RK, Thaler HT, et al: Pain and depression in patients with newly diagnosed pancreas cancer. J Clin Oncol 13:748–755, 1995

Kendall-Tackett KA: Physiological correlates of childhood abuse: chronic hyperarousal in PTSD, depression, and irritable bowel syndrome. Child Abuse Negl 24:799–810, 2000

Kim DY, Camilleri M: Serotonin: a mediator of the brain-gut connection. Am J Gastroenterol 95:2698–2709, 2000

Lee DH, Jamal H, Regenstein FG, et al: Morbidity of chronic hepatitis C as seen in a tertiary care medical center. Dig Dis Sci 42:186–191, 1997

Lee J, O'Morain C: Who should be treated for Helicobacter pylori infection? A review of consensus conferences and guidelines. Gastroenterology 113:S99–106, 1997

Lerner DM, Stoudemire A, Rosenstein DL: Neuropsychiatric toxicity associated with cytokine therapies. Psychosomatics 40:428–435, 1999

Levenstein S: The very model of a modern etiology: a biopsychosocial view of peptic ulcer. Psychosom Med 2:176–185, 2000

Levenstein S, Kaplan GA: Socioeconomic status and ulcer: a prospective study of contributory risk factors. J Clin Gastroenterol 26:14–17, 1998

Levenstein S, Prantera C, Varvo V, et al: Psychological stress and disease activity in ulcerative colitis: a multidimensional cross-sectional study. Am J Gastroenterol 89:1219–1225, 1994

Levy RL, Whitehead WE, Von Korff MR, et al: Intergenerational transmission of gastrointestinal illness behavior. Am J Gastroenterol 95:451–456, 2000

Leznoff A: Provocative challenges in patients with multiple chemical sensitivity. J Allergy Clin Immunol 99:438–442, 1997

Lipkin M, Lamb GS: The couvade syndrome: an epidemiologic study. Ann Intern Med 96:509–511, 1982

Locke GR, Zinsmeister AR, Talley NJ, et al: Risk factors for irritable bowel syndrome: role of analgesics and food sensitivities. Am J Gastroenterol 95:157–165, 2000

Lydiard RB, Fossey MD, Marsh W, et al: Prevalence of psychiatric disorders in patients with irritable bowel syndrome. Psychosomatics 34:229–234, 1993

Mayoral W, Lewis JH: Drug-induced liver disease. Curr Opin Gastroenterol 16:231–238, 2000

McDaniel JS, Musselman DL, Porter MR, et al: Depression in patients with cancer: diagnosis, biology and treatment. Arch Gen Psychiatry 52:89–99, 1995

McQuaid K: Dyspepsia, in Sleisenger and Fordtran's Gastrointestinal and Liver Disease, 6th Edition. Edited by Feldman M, Scharschmidt BF, Sleisenger MH, et al. Philadelphia, PA, WB Saunders, 1998, pp 105–115

Meggs WJ: Neurogenic switching: a hypothesis for a mechanism for shifting the site of inflammation in allergy and chemical sensitivity. Environ Health Perspect 103:54–56, 1995

Mertz H, Morgan V, Tanner G, et al: Regional cerebral activation in irritable bowel syndrome and control subjects with painful and non-painful rectal distention. Gastroenterology 118:842–848, 2000

Naliboff BD, Munakata J, Chang L, et al: Toward a biobehavioral model of visceral hypersensitivity in irritable bowel syndrome. J Psychosom Res 45:485–492, 1998

National Institutes of Health: National Institutes of Health Consensus Development Conference Panel Statement: management of hepatitis C. Hepatology 26 (3, suppl):2S–10S, 1997

North CS, Clouse RE, Spitznagel EL, et al: The relation of ulcerative colitis to psychiatric factors: a review of findings and methods. Am J Psychiatry 147:974–981, 1990

Noyes R, Cook B, Garvey M, et al: Reduction of gastrointestinal symptoms following treatment for panic disorder. Psychosomatics 31:75–79, 1990

Overmier JB, Murison R: Anxiety and helplessness in the face of stress predisposes, precipitates, and sustains gastric ulceration. Behav Brain Res 110:161–174, 2000

Panagiotis B: Grand mal seizures with liver toxicity in a case of clozapine treatment. J Neuropsychiatry Clin Neurosci 11:117–118, 1999

Passik SD, Breitbart WS: Depression in patients with pancreatic carcinoma: diagnostic and treatment issues. Cancer 78 (3 suppl):615–626, 1996

Passik SD, Roth AJ: Anxiety symptoms and panic attacks preceding pancreatic cancer diagnosis. Psychooncology 8:268–272, 1999

Payne A, Blanchard EB: A controlled comparison of cognitive therapy and self-help support groups in the treatment of irritable bowel syndrome. J Consult Clin Psychol 63:779–786, 1995

Petty F, Noyes R Jr: Depression secondary to cancer. Biol Psychiatry 16:1203–1220, 1981

Rask-Madsen C, Bresnick WH, Loss MA, et al: The effect of emotional stress on gastric acid secretion in normal subjects and duodenal ulcer patients [American Gastroenterological Association Abstracts]. Gastroenterology 98:A382, 1990

Richter JE: Noncardiac (unexplained) chest pain. Curr Treat Options Gastroenterol 3:329–334, 2000

Rigaud D, Bedig G, Merrouche M, et al: Delayed gastric emptying in anorexia nervosa is improved by completion of a renutrition program. Dig Dis Sci 33:919–925, 1988

Ringel Y, Drossman DA: Treatment of patients with functional esophageal symptoms: is there a role for a psychotherapeutic approach? J Clin Gastroenterol 28:189–193, 1999

Rix KJB, Pearson DF, Bentley SJ: A psychiatric study of patients with supposed food allergy. Br J Psychiatry 145:121–126, 1984

Ross BD, Danielsen ER, Bluml S: Proton magnetic resonance spectroscopy: the new gold standard for diagnosis of clinical and subclinical hepatic encephalopathy. Dig Dis 14 (suppl 1):30–39, 1996

Sarbah AS, Younossi ZM: Hepatitis C: an update on the silent epidemic. J Clin Gastroenterol 30:125–143, 2000

Schiff ER: Hepatitis C and alcohol. Hepatology 26 (3 suppl 1):39S–42S, 1997

Schuster MM: Care of patients with colostomy or ileostomy, in Principles of Ambulatory Medicine, 4th Edition. Edited by Barker LR, Burton JR, Zieve PD. Baltimore, MD, Williams & Wilkins, 1995, pp 468–472

Schwartz AI, Cole JO, Debattista CP: Manual of Clinical Psychopharmacology, 3rd Edition. Washington, DC, American Psychiatric Press, 1997, p 406

Selim K, Kaplowitz N: Hepatotoxicity of psychotropic drugs. Hepatology 29:1347–1351, 1999

Shen WW: The metabolism of psychoactive drugs: a review of enzymatic biotransformation and inhibition. Biol Psychiatry 41:814–826, 1997

Shorter E: Multiple chemical sensitivity: a pseudodisease in historical perspective. Scand J Work Environ Health 23 (suppl 3):35–42, 1997

Silverman DH, Munakata JA, Ennes H, et al: Regional cerebral activity in normal and pathological perception of visceral pain. Gastroenterology 112:64–72, 1997

Singh N, Gayowski T, Wagener MM, et al: Vulnerability to psychologic distress and depression in patients with end-stage liver disease due to hepatitis C virus. Clin Transplant 11:406–411, 1997

Singh N, Gayowski T, Wagener MM, et al: Quality of life, functional status, and depression in male liver transplant recipients with recurrent viral hepatitis C. Transplantation 67:69–72, 1999

Soll AH: Peptic ulcer and its complications, in Sleisenger and Fordtran's Gastrointestinal and Liver Disease, 6th Edition. Edited by Feldman M, Scharschmidt BF, Sleisenger MH, et al. Philadelphia, PA, WB Saunders, 1998, pp 621–669

Stenson WF: Inflammatory bowel disease, in Cecil Textbook of Medicine, 21st Edition. Edited by Goldman L, Bennett, JC. Philadelphia, PA, WB Saunders, 2000, pp 722–729

Stoudemire A, Moran M: Psychopharmacology in the medically ill, in The American Psychiatric Press Textbook of Psychopharmacology, 2nd Edition. Edited by Schatzberg AF, Nemeroff CB. Washington, DC, American Psychiatric Press, 1998, pp 931–960

Stoudemire A, Moran MG, Fogel BS: Psychotropic drug use in the medically ill, part II. Psychosomatics 32:34–46, 1991

Suarez FL, Savaiano D, Arbisi P, et al: Tolerance to the daily ingestion of two cups of milk by individuals claiming lactose intolerance. Am J Clin Nutr 65:1502–1506, 1997

Szigethy E, Wiznitzer M, Branicky LA, et al: Risperidone-induced hepatotoxicity in children and adolescents: a chart review study. J Child Adolesc Psychopharmacol 9:93–98, 1999

Talley NJ, Fung LH, Gilligan IJ, et al: Association of anxiety, neuroticism, and depression with dyspepsia of unknown cause. Gastroenterology 90:886–892, 1986

Talley NJ, Owen BK, Boyce P, et al: Psychological treatments for irritable bowel syndrome: a critique of controlled treatment trials. Am J Gastroenterol 91:277–286, 1996

Talley NJ, Stanghellini V, Heading RC, et al: Functional gastroduodenal disorders. Gut 45(suppl. II):II37–II42, 1999

Thompson WG, Longstreth GF, Drossman DA, et al: Functional bowel disorders and functional abdominal pain. Gut 45(suppl II):II43–II47, 1999

Trask PC, Esper P, Riba M, et al: Psychiatric side effects of interferon therapy: prevalence, proposed mechanisms, and future directions. J Clin Oncol 18:2316–2326, 2000

Valentine AD, Meyers CA, Kling MA, et al: Mood and cognitive side effects of interferon-alpha therapy. Semin Oncol 25 (suppl 1):39–47, 1998

Van der Rijt CC, Schalm SW, Meulstee J, et al: Flumazenil therapy for hepatic encephalopathy: a double-blind cross over study. Gastroenterol Clin Biol 19(6–7):572–580, 1995

Walker EA, Roy-Byrne PP, Katon WJ: Irritable bowel syndrome and psychiatric illness. Am J Psychiatry 147:565–572, 1990

Walker EA, Katon WJ, Roy-Byrne PP, et al: Histories of sexual victimization in patients with irritable bowel syndrome or inflammatory bowel disease. Am J Psychiatry 150:1502–1506, 1993

Walker EA, Gelfand AN, Gelfand MD, et al: Psychiatric diagnoses, sexual and physical victimization, and disability in patients with irritable bowel syndrome or inflammatory bowel disease. Psychol Med 25:1259–1267, 1995

Whitehead WE: Psychosocial aspects of functional gastrointestinal disorders. Gastroenterol Clin North Am 25:21–34, 1996

Whitehead WE, Holtkotter B, Enck P, et al: Tolerance for rectosigmoid distention in irritable bowel syndrome. Gastroenterology 98:1187–1192, 1990

Wise TN, Cooper JN, Ahmed S: The efficacy of group therapy for patients with irritable bowel syndrome. Psychosomatics 23:465–469, 1982

Woodman CL, Breen K, Noyes R, et al: The relationship between irritable bowel syndrome and psychiatric illness: a family study. Psychosomatics 39:45–54, 1998

Zabora J, BrintzenhofeSzoc K, Curbow B, et al: The prevalence of psychological distress by cancer site. Psychooncology 10:19–28, 2001

Chapter 3

Psychiatric Overview of Solid Organ Transplantation

Catherine C. Crone, M.D.
Geoffrey Gabriel, M.D.

In the twentieth century, the possibility of conquering end-stage organ disease and its grim prognosis transitioned from science fiction to fact with the advent of solid organ transplantation. Although early efforts were met with limited success, transplantation became a realistic treatment option after the introduction of cyclosporine in the 1970s. Since then, additional developments with immunosuppressant agents have resulted in greater success rates and a growing demand for donor organs. Currently, more than 75,000 patients await organ transplantation in the United States, which is more than triple the number of patients listed only a decade ago ("National organ transplant waiting list tops 75,000" 2001). Yearly, fewer than a third of patients receive a donor organ, and many die while on the organ transplant waiting list ("National organ transplant waiting list tops 75,000" 2001).

Patient Evaluation

Patients referred to transplant centers undergo multidisciplinary evaluations to determine whether they might benefit from receiving donor organs. Assessments include thorough history taking, physical examination, and several laboratory, radiological, and other diagnostic tests. Psychosocial evaluations for each candidate are also obtained. Review of this information allows transplant teams to select patients for placement on the donor organ waiting list.

Psychosocial information encompasses a wide range of non-medical issues pertaining to patients and their experiences (Dew et al. 2000b). This includes past and present psychiatric diagnoses, social support, treatment compliance, substance use, and cognitive capabilities. Prior experiences and response to health care providers, hospitalizations, and physical illness are also part of this database. Most transplant teams use psychosocial information when they consider patients for receipt of donor organs. However, programs differ in how the data are applied to their selection process. For example, some centers automatically turn down candidates with a history of recent suicide attempts, treatment noncompliance, or substance abuse (Levenson and Olbrisch 1993). Others will consider these patients on a case-by-case basis, whereas some will regard this information as irrelevant to their decision whether to list patients for transplantation (Levenson and Olbrisch 1993). Differences among centers in their perception of psychosocial information are affected by several factors, such as the type of organ being transplanted, the size of the program, and the level of experience with psychosocially complicated patients (Crone and Wise 1999b; Levenson and Olbrisch 2000).

Most programs rely on mental health professionals to perform psychosocial assessments on patients being considered for transplantation. Donor organ shortages combined with the high costs of transplantation spur teams to select patients whom they consider capable of achieving successful outcomes. Part of their decision making involves identification of candidates able to handle the uncertainties, demands, and setbacks inherent to organ transplantation. The ability to adhere to long-term medications, clinic visits, diagnostic tests, and other parts of post-transplant life is considered a necessity (Crone and Wise 1999b). Patients with limited coping skills, poor social support, self-destructive tendencies, or difficulties interacting with transplant team members are likely to be regarded as high-risk candidates (Levenson and Olbrisch 2000). Programs try to work with these individuals to determine whether problems can be overcome (Levenson and Olbrisch 1993). However, patients failing to respond to efforts will be removed from the waiting list or will not be offered listing in the first place.

In addition to their use in candidate selection, psychosocial assessments serve other purposes that affect both patients and transplant teams. Assessments foster the development of a working relationship between both parties and provide a time to inform patients and family members about the challenges ahead of them (Phipps 1991; Surman 1994). Awareness of these hurdles (i.e., indeterminate waiting time, postoperative complications, long-term medical care) allows patients and families to mobilize their abilities to work as a cohesive group (Phipps 1991; Surman 1994). Misunderstandings, unrealistic expectations, and underlying fears about transplantation also can be uncovered and addressed (Crone and Wise 1999b). Most important, psychosocial assessments allow teams to glimpse at their patients' strengths, weaknesses, and coping abilities (Fricchione 1989). Difficulties noted here can lead to early interventions and a chance to plan for the level of resources, care, and support that patients will need to undergo transplantation.

The psychosocial evaluation of transplant patients resembles the standard psychiatric interview, except for the addition of certain topics related to transplantation (Table 3–1). These include greater attention to the medical history, especially course of illness and compliance with office visits, invasive procedures, hospitalizations, and medications.

Table 3–1.	Pretransplant psychosocial evaluation
Current history	Cause of organ failure, course of illness, prior treatments, prior hospitalizations, current signs and symptoms, effect on daily functioning
Attitude toward and understanding of transplantation	Understands reasons for referral to transplant center; level of interest; expectations and concerns about transplantation; comprehension of risks, benefits, procedure, recovery

Table 3–1. Pretransplant psychosocial evaluation *(continued)*

Compliance	Both current and past compliance with medical follow-up, medications, tests, treatments (e.g., dialysis, pulmonary rehabilitation), dietary restrictions, fluid restrictions, abstinence from alcohol and tobacco
Past medical history	Prior illnesses other than organ failure, hospitalizations, operations, recovery experiences
Psychiatric history	Current or past disorders; illness severity; recurrences; prior experiences with mental health providers, hospitalizations, medications, response to treatment, compliance with treatment
Substance use or abuse	Alcohol, drugs, and tobacco—length of use, frequency of use, amount used, current use, reasons for abstinence (i.e., doctor's orders, too sick to tolerate being intoxicated), evidence of abuse or dependence
Family history	Medical, psychiatric, substance abuse
Social history	Particular attention placed on determining support system to care for patient if transplantation occurs; also, educational background, work history, current living situation, principal relationships, financial status, coping skills, concurrent stressors (e.g., primary caregiver for ill parent or child, legal problems)
Mental status	Emphasis on insight, judgment, attention, concentration, psychomotor retardation, short- or long-term memory

Patients also are asked about their interest in transplantation, their comprehension of its risks and benefits, and their motivation for pursuing this procedure (House and Thompson 1988; Olbrisch and Levenson 1995). An important consideration is informed consent because many patients have cognitive impairment from end-stage disease (Crone and Wise 1999b; Culledge et al. 1983). Neuropsychological testing may be required to determine whether patients can make reasonable decisions about transplantation (Tarter and Switala 2000). Although psychosocial evaluations are mostly obtained via unstructured interviews, standardized assessment tools are available to ensure that all relevant issues are covered. Both the Transplant Evaluation Rating Scale (TERS) and the Psychosocial Assessment of Candidates for Transplant (PACT) have been validated and show good interrater reliability (Olbrisch et al. 1989; Twillman et al. 1993). Although the Structured Interview for Renal Transplantation (SIRT) still needs validation, it is one more option to assist in the pretransplant evaluation (Mori et al. 2000).

Problematic Patients: Noncompliance

Successful posttransplant outcomes depend on several factors, including compliance with daily medications, laboratory tests, clinic appointments, biopsies, self-measurements, and lifestyle modifications. Studies of posttransplant patients found noncompliance rates ranging from 20% to 60%, with the highest rates seen in younger patients and adolescents (Bunzel and Laederach-Hoffman 2000). Although noncompliance does not always result in complications, it is a frequent cause of acute and chronic rejection, as well as graft failure (Dew and Kormos 1999; Douglas et al. 1996; Gaston et al. 1999). Compliance also tends to decline over time, even among patients who are initially compliant (Dew et al. 2000b). Because noncompliance may not respond to corrective measures, transplant teams have focused on identifying patients at highest risk for this behavior (Haynes et al. 1996).

Although researchers have tried to predict which patients will become noncompliant, their efforts have remained unsuccessful (Bunzel and Laederach-Hoffman 2000). Nonetheless, studies have been able to detect some patient characteristics associated with noncompliance. Educational level, sex, and racial/ethnic background have been correlated with noncompliance in several, but not all, studies (De Geest et al. 1998; Gaston et al. 1999; Siegel and Greenstein 1997). Stronger connections have been found between noncompliance and adolescence, as well as length of time since transplantation (Bunzel and Laederach-

Hoffman 2000; Dew et al. 2000b; Greenstein and Siegal 1998). Dew and colleagues (1996b), Chacko et al. (1996b), and Shapiro et al. (1995) also noted connections between noncompliance and anxiety, depression, hostility, substance abuse, personality disorder, and avoidant coping style. Another factor to be considered is a history of noncompliance because this tends to recur posttransplantation (Douglas et al. 1996; Olbrisch and Levenson 1995). In general, these variables should not exclude patients from transplantation; rather, they should alert teams to patients in need of closer attention and care. Additional efforts made before transplantation, such as establishing stable social support, can allow many of these patients to undergo successful transplantation (Chacko et al. 1996a).

Problematic Patients: Substance Abuse

Alcohol is one of the most common causes of end-stage liver disease in the United States and is not infrequently a risk factor among cases of cardiomyopathy (DiMartini and Trzepacz 2000). Alcoholic cirrhosis develops in only a relatively small portion of patients with alcohol dependence, and some will develop cirrhosis without meeting DSM-IV-TR (American Psychiatric Association 2000) criteria for alcohol abuse or dependence (DiMartini and Trzepacz 2000). Providing transplantation to patients with substance-induced organ disease has long been an area of dispute between the public, ethicists, and health care providers (Moss and Siegler 1991; Schenker et al. 1990). Discussion has mainly centered on liver transplantation for alcoholic cirrhosis because this is the second leading indication for this procedure. There is clearly concern over the concept of organs being given to those with self-induced disease, yet most overlook the fact that alcoholism is not a moral failure but a disease unto itself. Transplant teams have also wrestled over transplanting those with alcohol-induced liver disease, but initial concerns about survival and outcome have not been justified by subsequent results (Hoofnagle et al. 1997; Pageaux et al. 1999).

Because patients with alcoholic cirrhosis have done well with transplantation, most centers have shifted their attention to the problem of relapse. This is partially because of studies that have

---

found a correlation between alcohol relapse and greater medical complications (Campbell and Punch 1997; Pereira and Williams 1997). These complications are thought to be a result of the toxic effects of alcohol on bodily tissues and/or the emergence of non-compliant behaviors (Abosh et al. 2000; Pereira and Williams 1997; Shapiro et al. 1995). Recent studies have reported a much higher incidence of relapse posttransplant than was originally thought to exist (Abosh et al. 2000; Everson et al. 1997; Gerhardt et al. 1998; Pageaux et al. 1999). Thus, transplant programs have tried to find ways to reduce the likelihood of relapse among patients with alcohol-related liver disease. A common approach involves the 6-month abstinence rule that was based on earlier findings linking length of abstinence to relapse rates (Kumar et al. 1990). Subsequent research has yielded mixed results, with several studies noting no association between a 6-month period of abstinence pretransplant and relapse posttransplantation (Gerhardt et al. 1998; Tringali et al. 1996).

Rather than rely on a mandatory period of abstinence, many have argued for the use of alternative predictors of relapse. These tend to be derived from studies involving nontransplant alcoholic populations. For example, Beresford et al. (1990) and Vaillant et al. (1983) used results from long-term abstinence studies to develop prognostic factors for liver transplant candidates. These include acceptance of the diagnosis of dependence, social stability, sources of hope or self-esteem, and noxious consequences for relapse (Beresford et al. 1990). Yates et al. (1993) applied another group of factors to derive his High-Risk Alcoholism Relapse Scale, which has been undergoing study in liver transplant patients (DiMartini et al. 2000). Unfortunately, there are still no variables that can reliably predict posttransplant relapse (DiMartini and Trzepacz 2000). Instead, some centers have decided to emphasize the treatment of addictive behaviors. Patients may be required to attend Alcoholics Anonymous or Narcotics Anonymous meetings or complete formal rehabilitation programs. Behavioral contracts can be added to reinforce treatment requirements (Everhart and Beresford 1997; Nelson et al. 1995). Only those fulfilling requirements go on to receive transplants.

An issue needing further attention is the evaluation of transplant candidates enrolled in methadone maintenance programs. This may be of greater concern because of the growing number of patients with hepatitis C–induced liver failure needing transplantation (G.L. Davis 2000). Few reports have been published about transplanting these patients, but outcomes appear to be positive (Gordon et al. 1986; Koch and Banys 2001). Many centers have difficulty distinguishing methadone maintenance from opioid dependence, as reflected in results from a recent survey (Koch and Banys 2001). Nearly half of the liver transplant teams polled would not accept candidates receiving methadone maintenance, and a third would require discontinuation of methadone before transplantation (Koch and Banys 2001). This view is clearly at odds with findings from methadone maintenance research and likely sets up this population for relapse posttransplantation (Joseph et al. 2000; Koch and Banys 2001). Thus, centers need education and help from mental health professionals to avoid discrimination.

Problematic Patients: Axis I and II Disorders

In addition to problems with substance abuse, other forms of psychiatric illness are not uncommon among patients presenting for transplant evaluation. Studies of those with end-stage organ disease, some referred for transplantation, indicate high rates of anxiety and depression (Goldberg and Posner 2000; McDaniel et al. 2000; Thompson 2000). Often, these are in the form of major depression or panic and adjustment disorders (Freeman et al. 1988; Trumper and Appleby 2001). Personality disorders also have been detected during transplant assessments, either alone or accompanying an Axis I disorder (Dobbels et al. 2000). Psychological distress is likely to be tied to losses in physical health, independence, functional abilities, social stability, and financial resources. Medications used to manage organ disease also can produce signs and symptoms of depression, anxiety, or personality changes (Goldberg and Posner 2000; Levenson and Dwight 2000; Thompson 2000). Similar difficulties also may appear as a result of hepatic, hypoxic, or uremic encephalopathy (Rodin and

Abbey 1992; Thompson 2000; Trzepacz et al. 1989).

Transplant centers have long sought to select candidates who are capable of coping with the long-term demands and stressors of transplantation. Early reports implied that those with psychiatric disorders were prone to develop noncompliance and poor quality of life following transplantation (Brennan et al. 1987; Surman 1989). Subsequent experiences have been mixed, with many having good outcomes (Woodman et al. 1999; Yates et al. 1998). Current findings support the need to individualize patient assessments. This calls for careful history taking, with attention to behaviors, attitudes, or symptoms that could interfere with the task of adjusting to transplantation. Complete information provides teams with the foresight to plan needed psychosocial interventions and to determine whether they have resources available to work with these patients.

Certain patient populations with psychiatric disorders create significant unease among transplant programs. One of these is psychotic patients, whether due to bipolar disorder, schizophrenia, or other illnesses. This group is most at risk for being turned down for transplantation, especially if active symptoms are present (Levenson and Olbrisch 1993). Unfortunately, this rejection comes without clear distinction of the particular signs and symptoms factoring into poor outcomes. Only a few cases have been published regarding transplantation in psychotic patients, and one study examined individual patient variables (Coffman and Crone 1999; DiMartini and Twillman 1994). Results from this study indicated that living alone, being homeless, or having positive psychotic symptoms within the year before being transplanted was associated with a five to six times greater incidence of immunosuppressant noncompliance and suicide attempts (Coffman and Crone 1999).

Another group causing apprehension is composed of patients presenting in acute liver failure from intentional acetaminophen overdoses. This is the primary cause of acute liver failure in both the United States and the United Kingdom (Fontana and Quallich 2001). Fortunately, most patients recover and do not need transplantation, but a few will progress to this stage. Assessing overdose patients for transplantation can be affected by team biases or overidentification with patients and family members (Aulisio and Arnold 1996; Forster et al. 1996). This adds to the need for objective psychosocial evaluations by mental health professionals. Careful interview of family members and other sources of collateral information are vital. This is especially important if patients are already comatose when seen. Issues that need to be covered include contributing factors leading to the attempt, receptiveness to psychiatric treatment posttransplantation, availability of social support, history of attempts, and attitude toward transplantation (i.e., wants to live?) (Greiner 1990). After gathering the data, mental health professionals can convey this information to transplant teams and assist them in making an unbiased decision.

Pretransplant Waiting Period

The period leading from evaluation to transplantation is defined by multiple psychological, medical, and social stresses with the potential to cause widespread complications (Craven 1989; House and Thompson 1988). The role of the psychiatrist in the pretransplant period is to assist the patient, family members, and transplant team as they work to navigate individual and group issues. Certain medical and psychological trends should be anticipated, recognized, and treated to maximize the functional status of the patient in the pretransplant period (Surman 1994).

Psychological Issues

The pretransplant period is marked by numerous conflicting psychological demands on the patient and family (Hickey and Leske 1992; Kuhn et al. 1990). Being placed on the transplant list is often met initially with a sense of renewed hope and optimism that collides with the continued threat of death should the patient's condition decline before organ availability. The length of time from being listed to being transplanted is dictated by a host of variables, most of which are out of the control of the patient and his or her family (Collins et al. 1996; Nolan et al. 1992).

Patients who are receiving organs from a cadaveric source often feel guilty. The fact that one life must end so that another life can continue is a harsh reality the patient is forced to process. Some patients become preoccupied with fantasies surrounding the personal characteristics of the donor, his or her survivors, and the form of death. Guilt may be heightened when the patient feels that his or her end-stage organ failure was caused directly by previous personal habits such as alcohol consumption or poor medical compliance.

During the pretransplant period, dependency is a major issue. Those with a preexisting dependent character structure may become increasingly passive and regressive. They are often unable to make rudimentary decisions and may cause frustration and alienation among teams and family members (House et al. 1983). The patient whose dependency needs are not met may become hostile toward the health care team, especially if the patient has idealized them.

Feelings of competitiveness are often mixed with the emotions of mistrust and empathy during the pretransplant period (Levenson and Olbrisch 1987). Patients closely follow the clinical situation of other listed patients, finding hope when a successful transplant occurs; however, ruminations of priority, favoritism, and connections may be expressed in a hostile or entitled manner by the patients who remain on the list (Levenson and Olbrisch 1987). Should the transplanted patient's condition worsen and organ failure occur, self-recrimination and guilt may be expressed openly or defensively projected onto others in the patient's environment. When competitiveness becomes an organizing theme for the patient, the benefits of mutual support from other patients are often lost.

Denial has often been overcome by the time the patient has been placed on the waiting list. Acceptance of the fact that end-organ failure is likely a terminal state fluctuates with varying degrees of intellectualization and isolation of affect. Ambivalence may occur when patients begin to closely examine the reality of the quality of life following transplant. The ambivalent patient may express a desire to be transplanted while acting in ways that compromise function and status. Ambivalence that is not fully detected and addressed in the pretransplant period likely places the patient at risk for suboptimal outcome in the posttransplant period.

The pretransplant period presents the debilitated patient with certain developmental tasks that may increase psychological morbidity (Levenson and Olbrisch 1987). He or she faces a decreased quality of life associated with physical infirmity and the loss of a body that was once competent. The loss of strength, pleasure, and agility once derived from an intact body may be met with feelings of despair, anger, and disappointment. This is especially significant if the patient is forced to deal with a decline in sexual activity secondary to medical constraints.

The development of roles and relationships often collide in the pretransplant period, resulting in frustration, perplexity, and amazement (Collins et al. 1996). The manner in which the patient processes this milestone is dependent on the integration of prior significant relationships in the area of love, occupation, and society. A reversal of roles often occurs when the patient must relinquish control of certain aspects of his or her life to others (Buse and Pieper 1990; Jalowiec et al. 1994). If this is met with a sense of surrender, despair and depression are likely outcomes. The patient also may begin to reestablish (and often rework) former relationships while expanding the capacity to forge new ties, especially with members of the transplant team.

Depression

Depression is common during the pretransplant period regardless of the type of organ to be transplanted (Benning and Smith 1994; F. Mai 1993; Surman 1994; Trzpacz et al. 1989). Because of its many possible presentations in this patient population, detection often may be difficult. Complicating factors include symptoms and signs produced by medications or physiological conditions (DiMartini and Trzepacz 1999). Stated dysphoric mood, cognitions of hopelessness and helplessness, a sense of demoralization, and active or passive suicidal ideation warrant rapid evaluation and treatment. Additional clues to a depressive episode may include a decrease in the patient's active participation in his or her medical care, reversal of the patient's decision to be transplanted, failure to adhere to medical or lifestyle regimens, or a change in the patient's perception of his or her health status. Collateral data from team members, family, and other social supports are often vital in detecting a depressive episode in the pretransplant patient.

Pharmacological treatment of depression in the pretransplant patient mandates careful consideration of altered physiological parameters resulting from particular end-stage organ failure (Table 3–2). In addition, drug-drug interactions and effects of a particular medication on the cytochrome P450 enzymes must be considered (Brown et al. 2000; DiMartini and Trzepacz 1999). The selective serotonin reuptake inhibitors (SSRIs) usually are well tolerated in the medically ill pretransplant patient because of their low incidence of antihistaminic or anticholinergic side effects. SSRIs generally are free of cardiotoxic effects, including conduction abnormalities, changes in blood pressure, and increases in heart rate (Tollefson and Rosenbaum 1998). Elimination half-lives of SSRIs are increased in the context of phase I (reduction, oxidation, hydrolysis) hepatic metabolism dysfunction that occurs with hepatitis and cirrhosis (Dalhoff et al. 1991; Demolis et al. 1996). Adjustments in dosing may be necessary in renal dysfunction and dialysis. Interactions of the SSRIs with the various cytochrome P450 enzymes, especially inhibition, should be considered following a through review of the patient's medication profile.

Bupropion also can be considered a first-line treatment for pretransplant depression, especially for patients presenting with apathy and amotivational components. It appears to have minimal significant adverse cardiovascular effects, even in overdose (Kiev et al. 1994; Roose et al. 1991; Spiller et al. 1994). However, bupropion should be used cautiously with patients who have a lowered seizure threshold, especially when encephalopathy is present (Strouse et al. 1993).

Nefazodone has side effects and interactions that limit its use for the pretransplant patient. It has significant inhibition of the cytochrome P450 3A4 enzymes, which serve to metabolize numerous medications used in transplant patients, including dihydropyridine calcium channel blockers, antirejection medications, analgesics, and angiotensin-converting enzyme inhibitors

Table 3–2. Antidepressants: considerations in end-stage organ disease

Medication	Starting dose (mg/day)	Comments/side effects
Fluoxetine	10–20	Inhibits cytochrome P450 2D6; may increase levels of haloperidol; no effect on levels of cyclosporine; risk of syndrome of inappropriate secretion of antidiuretic hormone; reduce dose in hepatic disease
Paroxetine	10–20	Potent inhibitor of cytochrome P450 2D6; considered mildly anticholinergic; no cardiac effects; mild sedation
Sertraline	25–50	Possible sinus bradycardia; minimal inhibition of cytochrome P450 2D6; may increase levels of warfarin; less likely to cause extrapyramidal side effects
Citalopram	10–20	Prolonged half-life in hepatic disease; Q-Tc prolongation in overdose; metabolized by cytochrome P450 3A4 and 2C19
Fluvoxamine	25–50	Short half-life; increased levels of warfarin; inhibits cytochrome P450 3A4 and 1A2; increased levels of haloperidol
Bupropion	75–100	Seizure risk; minimal cardiac effects; useful for apathetic/amotivational symptoms; may induce agitation or psychosis; minimal P450 effects; sustained formulation available
Nefazodone	50–100	Potent inhibitor of cytochrome P450 3A4; sedating; metabolite (m-chlorophenylpiperazine) can cause anxiety symptoms; may cause orthostatic hypotension

Table 3–2. Antidepressants: considerations in end-stage organ disease *(continued)*

Medication	Starting dose (mg/day)	Comments/side effects
Venlafaxine	37.5–75	Dose-dependent increase in blood pressure; sedating; minimal protein binding; half-life increased in hepatic and renal disease
Mirtazapine	7.5–15	Minimal P450 effects; anxiolytic, sedative qualities; agranulocytosis and hyperlipidemia rare; minimal cardiac effects

(Greene and Barbhaiya 1997; Vella and Sayegh 1998). In addition, levels of the parent compound and metabolite (*m*-chlorophenylpiperazine [m-CPP]) are increased in patients with hepatic cirrhosis; however, no dose reduction is apparently required with renal impairment (Barbhaiya et al. 1995; Brown and Stoudemire 1998). Anxiety has been associated with increased levels of m-CPP (Cunningham et al. 1994).

Venlafaxine may be particularly useful in depressed pretransplant patients with significant anxiety. Venlafaxine appears to have no cardiotoxicity, but it can increase blood pressure in a dose-related manner (Cunningham et al. 1994). Because of decreased clearance, dosing will need to be modified in patients with cirrhosis or renal impairment.

The specific receptor blockade of mirtazapine produces anxiolytic effects while promoting sleep and appetite (de Boer 1996). Blockade of the serotonin type 3 receptors may decrease medication-induced nausea. Weight gain and its associated medical complications are possible side effects, but the use of mirtazapine has not been associated with heart rate or blood pressure changes (Montgomery 1995). Because of its sedative qualities, mirtazapine should be used with caution in those patients prone to delirium. Dosing also should be reduced in patients with hepatic disease (Beliles and Stoudemire 1998).

Anxiety

Anxiety, whether as a component of a depressive disorder or as a unique disorder, is prevalent during the pretransplant period (Benning and Smith 1994; Deshields et al. 1996). Multiple factors, including medication side effects; metabolic, respiratory, and endocrine dysregulation; poor pain control; and psychosocial stresses, can contribute to the development of anxiety (Smoller et al. 1996; Woodman et al. 1999). Unrecognized or inadequately treated anxiety may be associated with increased medical complications and suicide risk in the medically ill patient (Beautrais 2001; Kim et al. 2000; Mayou et al. 2000; Stoudemire 1996).

Benzodiazepines, especially those with short half-lives and no active metabolites, are useful in the treatment of anxiety in the pretransplant patient. The most commonly used include lorazepam, oxazepam, and clonazepam, with the latter having the longest half-life. Lorazepam is particularly useful because it has multiple routes of administration. Those such as diazepam, alprazolam, and chlordiazepoxide that rely on oxidation for biotransformation should be avoided in the medically ill pretransplant patient. In patients with liver disease, benzodiazepine use should be limited because of the potential for worsening preexisting encephalopathy (Bakti et al. 1987).

Buspirone is an attractive alternative to the use of benzodiazepines when the anxiety condition is not acute or overwhelming for the patient. It does not significantly induce or inhibit the cytochrome P450 system and has few side effects. Buspirone does not negatively affect respiratory function, is not cardiotoxic, and does not produce psychomotor impairment that may occur with the benzodiazepines (Garner et al. 1989). Major drawbacks of buspirone use include delayed onset of action and possible elevation of cyclosporine levels (Ninan et al. 1998). Buspirone also requires a dose reduction in the presence of renal dysfunction and may not be as effective in patients who have been exposed to extensive benzodiazepine use (DeMarinis et al. 2000; DeVane 1990).

The use of the various antidepressants in the treatment of anxiety in the pretransplant patient should be considered when the benzodiazepines are contraindicated. The SSRIs, venlafaxine, and mirtazapine may be useful in the treatment of anxiety disorders (Papp et al. 1998; Pohl et al. 1998; Rickels et al. 1993). In addition to pharmacotherapy, various relaxation techniques, hypnosis, and cognitive-behavioral therapy can be used.

Medical Issues

Delirium, often with multiple etiologies, is a common complication in the pretransplant period. End-stage organ failure may produce delirium through toxic substances that are not effectively removed or by decreased delivery of substances such as glucose and oxygen to the brain (Hazell and Butterworth 1999). In addition, delirium is often iatrogenic secondary to multiple medications or procedures such as dialysis. Hepatic, cardiac, and renal failure may individually or synergistically result in the development of delirium.

Hepatic encephalopathy may be acute in cases in which liver failure is secondary to hepatitis or toxic overdose. This condition often is associated with rapid progression to coma, increased central nervous system edema and intracranial pressure, and brain stem herniation (Clemmensen et al. 1999; Hazell and Butterworth 1999). Portosystemic encephalopathy, associated with portal hypertension and cirrhosis, typically has a slower progression that is often initially marked by personality or mood changes (E. Jones and Weissenborn 1997). In addition, patients with cirrhosis may have a subclinical type of hepatic encephalopathy without specific neurocognitive changes (Quero and Schalm 1996).

Multiple neurotransmitter systems, including γ-aminobutyric acid (GABA) and glutamate, are affected in hepatic encephalopathy (Hazell and Butterworth 1999). Ammonia may increase GABAergic tone and decrease the reuptake of glutamate by astrocytes (Norenberg et al. 1997). The decreased reuptake of glutamate by astrocytes results in a decrease in N-methyl-D-aspartate (NMDA) receptors (Michalak and Butterworth 1997). The combination of decreased glutamate neurotransmission and increased GABAergic tone may partially explain the neuroinhibitory symptoms associated with hepatic encephalopathy.

Psychiatric sequelae of hepatic encephalopathy can present with a multitude of symptoms ranging from irritability to hallucinations and delusions. The psychotic symptoms can be managed with low-dose haloperidol in conjunction with standard treatments for encephalopathy, including diet, lactulose, and antibiotic treatment. Experience is limited with the atypical antipsychotics in the treatment of hepatic encephalopathy. Because of the lack of studies, the routine use of flumazenil to reverse symptoms associated with hepatic encephalopathy cannot be recommended at this time (Cadranel et al. 1995; Gry et al. 1996).

Social Issues

The pretransplant period presents numerous social stresses on the patient and his or her support systems. Being placed on the transplant list brings with it a multitude of restrictions and forced adaptations on areas such as vocation or occupation, social performance, family relationships, residence, and finances (Gross et al. 1999; Levenson and Olbrisch 1987). Many of these aspects are explored in quality-of-life studies that examine physical, mental, and social parameters during the pre- and posttransplant periods (Rosenblum et al. 1993).

Where the patient resides while awaiting transplant varies with considerations such as medical condition, location of the transplant center, status on the transplant list, and support systems. Even patients who are able to remain at home feel constrained by not being able to travel or make long-term plans. Those who are hospitalized while awaiting transplant may be separated from family or other support systems because of the expense of relocation to a distant transplant center. The effect of separation from family varies depending on the age of the patient.

Often, the chronic end-stage illness that has brought the patient to the point of requiring transplantation has caused forced retirement, leading to a decline in self-esteem, the loss of sense of purpose, and feelings of isolation. For those who become ill near retirement or after retirement, plans for leisure and personal enhancement are interrupted.

Financial and economic solvencies are major psychosocial stresses in the pretransplant period. Interruption in a caregiver's ability to work because of time spent in the care of the patient or the need for relocation can cause significant financial hardships. Depending on insurance coverage, the patient and family are often faced with mounting medical bills that threaten to deplete their financial resources. The patient may begin to feel that he or she is a financial burden on his or her family and their future.

Perioperative Period

The challenge of surviving the waiting period is rewarded by the news that a donor organ is available. This knowledge gives renewed hope to patients and families but also means new challenges. Often, the first hurdle is the initial recovery from transplant surgery, with most patients beginning in the intensive care unit. Difficulties appear as neuropsychiatric disturbances that can cause excessive morbidity, mortality, and suffering if left untreated. Psychiatrists can play an active role in this setting by working with patients, families, and hospital staff.

Intensive Care Unit Environment

For most transplant recipients, the perioperative period will be their first experience with the intensive care unit setting. Patients awaken from anesthesia and find themselves in a foreign environment, surrounded by unfamiliar caregivers, sights, and sounds. Those on mechanical ventilation will be unable to communicate their questions, concerns, and needs to staff (Crone and Wise 1999a). Discomfort from being intubated and having a machine force breaths into one's lungs can be particularly disturbing (Boland et al. 2000; Crone and Wise 1999a). Pain may come from surgical wounds or long periods of immobility. Movement is restricted by monitors, catheters, and intravenous lines. Reassurance from family or friends is limited to brief periods, leaving patients isolated in this setting. Because of noises, lighting, discomfort, and constant activity, needed rest can be nearly impossible. Delirium will heighten the negative qualities of the intensive care unit. Psychiatrists can help the staff to reduce the potential for confusion and distress by suggesting simple environmental alterations (Boland et al. 2000; Meagher 2001) (Table 3–3).

Table 3–3. Intensive care unit environmental changes to reduce distress and confusion

Provide clock, calendar, daily schedule, and familiar items (photographs) to facilitate orientation. Ask staff and visitors to help reorient patient throughout the day.

Check with patient or family to determine whether glasses or hearing aids are normally used. Continued use in the intensive care unit can reduce tendency to misinterpret surroundings.

Use radios or televisions to provide sensory stimulation, but keep them at low volumes and ensure nonviolent content.

Dim room and minimize procedures and tasks during the evening to simulate day-night cycle.

Provide prompt correction if patient misinterprets environment (e.g., intravenous pole=person standing in the room). Do not challenge beliefs if patient is already delusional.

Provide alphabet board or develop alternative method of communication (e.g., blink eyes or raise finger to signal yes or no) if patient cannot verbalize needs or concerns.

Use relaxation training and hypnosis to reduce anxiety or stress caused by immobility or mechanical ventilation.

Ensure adequate pain control, administer medications on regularly scheduled basis, and refrain from use of as-needed dosing.

Provide clear, simple information about medical care and upcoming procedures or tests to help patient maintain some sense of control.

If delirium develops, educate family about the condition and reassure them that patient is not "going crazy." Provide reassurance to patient when delirium clears.

Neuropsychiatric Effects of Immunosuppressants

Immunosuppressant agents are necessary to reduce the body's ability to reject a donor organ. Cyclosporine and tacrolimus are the principal medications used; both work at the level of T lymphocytes. They are used on a long-term basis, starting with higher doses and tapering over time. Rejection episodes may be treated with increased doses or the addition of other immunosuppressants. Patients usually are maintained on one of these agents, along with a combination of steroids, azathioprine, or mycophenolate mofetil. Newer drugs also appear on a regular basis.

Although tacrolimus and cyclosporine are effective immuno-suppressants, they can cause a variety of neuropsychiatric complications. These tend to materialize within the first few days or weeks after transplantation, often when recipients are in the perioperative phase. Symptoms can emerge at therapeutic drug levels and may be accompanied by white matter changes on head computed tomography or magnetic resonance imaging scans (Hauben 1996; Singh et al. 2000). Liver and lung recipients seem to be more susceptible to neuropsychiatric problems (Craven and Toronto Lung Transplant Group 1990; De Groen and Craven 1992). Most resolve after dosage reductions over the course of several days. In some cases, resolution may take weeks or months, with rare cases of permanent complications.

The incidence of cyclosporine neurotoxicity ranges from 10% to 25%, generally appearing as tremor, headache, insomnia, restlessness, anxiety, blurred vision, apathy, and paresthesia (Craven and Toronto Lung Transplant Group 1990; De Groen and Craven 1992; Guarino et al. 1996; Hauben 1996; Miller 1996; Singh et al. 2000; Trzepacz 2000). Less common but more severe are seizures, delirium, psychosis, paresis, akinetic mutism, spasticity, dysarthria, cortical blindness, cerebral abscess, or coma (Adams et al. 1987; Trzepacz 2000; Valldeoriola et al. 1996). Neurotoxicity occurs more frequently when cyclosporine levels increase rapidly or fluctuate widely (Adams et al. 1987). Variables thought to predispose to cyclosporine complications include fever, infection, intravenous administration, high-dose steroids, hypomagnesemia, hypocholesterolemia, and previous hepatic encephalopathy or advanced liver failure (Adams et al. 1987; de Groen et al. 1987, 1989; Miller 1996). Neuropsychiatric difficulties linked to tacrolimus are very similar to those caused by cyclosporine (Bronster et al. 2000; Eidelman et al. 1991). However, tacrolimus may have a greater tendency to cause severe neuropsychiatric complications (McDiarmid et al. 1995).

Despite evidence pointing to tacrolimus and cyclosporine, corticosteroids are frequently blamed for neuropsychiatric symptoms noted among transplant recipients. Steroids are commonly used as part of the immunosuppressant regimen but may cause problems in only 5%–6% of patients (Kershner and Wang-Cheng

1989; Lewis and Smith 1983). Anxiety, distractibility, insomnia, depression, sensory flooding, mania, psychosis, and delirium all have been reported (Hall et al. 1979; Kershner and Wang-Cheng 1989; Lewis and Smith 1983). More often, patients have mild to moderate mood changes, particularly irritability (Lewis and Smith 1983).

Contrary to concerns, patients with current psychiatric disorders and those with a history of steroid psychosis are not more prone to steroid-induced difficulties (Kershner and Wang-Cheng 1989). High doses of steroids used early in the postoperative course and during rejection episodes may increase the odds of neuropsychiatric problems (Boston Collaborative Drug Surveillance Program 1972). Typically, symptoms are transient, although they may require treatment with psychotropic medications (Lewis and Smith 1983).

Mycophenolate mofetil and OKT3 are additional immunosuppressant drugs used by transplant programs. Both agents can aid in the treatment of refractory rejection, and mycophenolate mofetil also can be used as a standard immunosuppressant. Aseptic meningitis is the most frequent neuropsychiatric complication related to OKT3 (Trzepacz 2000). Other difficulties, including cerebral edema, cerebritis, seizures, delirium, tremor, and coma, are unusual (Trzepacz 2000). Mycophenolate mofetil has a low incidence of side effects, but tremors, insomnia, anxiety, depression, hypertonia, paresthesias, and somnolence have been reported (Trzepacz 2000).

Delirium

Delirium is a common problem during the perioperative period and requires prompt attention to avoid unnecessary morbidity and mortality. Critical care staff often use the term *intensive care unit psychosis* when referring to delirious patients, but this is a serious misnomer (McGuire et al. 2000). Patients who are labeled as such are believed to be cognitively impaired solely as a result of the effects of sleep and sensory deprivation (Wise and Trzepacz 1996). This concept interferes with the necessary evaluation and treatment of factors responsible for causing delirium.

Diagnosis and Screening

Delirium is characterized by altered consciousness, cognitive changes, and perceptual disturbances that tend to fluctuate over any given 24-hour period (American Psychiatric Association 2000). Symptoms or signs develop over a short period of time and tend to wax and wane in severity (American Psychiatric Association 2000). Inspecting nursing assessments across several shifts can help to expose cognitive and behavioral fluctuations (Liptzkin 2000). The same patients may be described as agitated or sluggish, demanding or cooperative, leading to a confusing picture. Problems often appear in the evenings because delirium often causes day-night reversals (Crone and Wise 1999a). Hallucinations and delusions may be seen and frequently are of paranoid content. Delirium can mimic any psychiatric disorder, so it should be considered when patients are described as anxious, depressed, manic, hostile, or psychotic. Information from family or friends about a patient's baseline personality also helps in discerning whether cognitive or behavioral changes are present.

Part of the task of caring for transplant recipients perioperatively involves helping staff to preidentify patients at higher risk for delirium so that they can be closely monitored (Crone and Wise 1999a). Patients who are elderly or have preexisting cognitive impairment (e.g., hepatic or hypoxic encephalopathy) are especially prone to delirium (Litaker et al. 2001). Early episodes of rejection that call for use of higher doses of immunosuppressants also place patients at risk (Strouse et al. 1996b; Trzepacz et al. 1991). Concurrent renal impairment and low serum albumin impair metabolism and clearance of drugs, also raising the risk for delirium (Levy 1990; Trzepacz and Francis 1990).

Causative Factors

Among transplant recipients, delirium is often multifactorial in origin. Patients typically are taking several medications other than immunosuppressant agents that can cause mental status changes (Abramowicz 1998; Liptzkin 2000) (Table 3–4). Overlapping drugs used to relieve pain, induce sleep, and reduce restlessness also can produce delirium (Crone and Wise 1999a).

Because patients are immunosuppressed after transplantation, infections from bacterial, fungal, and viral organisms also need to be considered (Rabkin et al. 2000; Selby et al. 1997). Metabolic imbalance and hypoxia also are potential causes of mental status changes (Liptzkin 2000). Neurological complications from cerebral hemorrhage or central pontine myelinolysis are unusual but should be considered if focal signs are present or other causes of delirium have already been ruled out (Wang et al. 2000; Wijdicks et al. 1996).

Table 3–4. Medications contributing to delirium onset

Immunosuppressants	Cyclosporine, tacrolimus, corticosteroids, mycophenolate mofetil, OKT3
Narcotics	Morphine sulfate, codeine, hydromorphone, hydrocodone, oxycodone, propoxyphene
Sedatives-hypnotics	Benzodiazepines, zolpidem, zaleplon, diphenhydramine
Cardiovascular drugs	Calcium channel blockers, angiotensin-converting enzyme inhibitors, β-blockers, misoprostol (prostaglandin E1)
Gastrointestinal drugs	Omeprazole, ranitidine, famotidine, metoclopramide, prochlorperazine, promethazine
Antibiotics, antivirals, antifungals	Cephalosporins, imipenem, penicillins, quinolones, sulfonamides, ganciclovir, acyclovir, foscarnet

Management

Psychiatrists often are asked to assist in the management of patients who have become agitated, confused, or combative in the intensive care unit. Most of these patients are delirious and require appropriate sedation. Neuroleptics remain the primary choice because they provide both sedation and a reduction in cognitive impairment (Boland et al. 2000; Tesar and Stern 1986). Even at higher doses, they have little effect on cardiovascular or respiratory functions (Boland et al. 2000; Fish 1991). In most cases, use of high-potency agents is preferred because they have few anticholinergic effects. The atypical antipsychotic agents are another choice, but limited data are available on their use in the hospital setting (Furmaga et al. 1997; Sipahimalani and Masand 1998).

Both haloperidol and droperidol have proven to be effective in the intensive care unit, but droperidol tends to produce more hypotension (Beliles 2000). Haloperidol is more flexible because it can be given intravenously, intramuscularly, or orally. The intravenous route may be preferable because of the lower frequency of extrapyramidal side effects (Menza et al. 1987). Initial doses start at 0.5–10 mg, depending on the degree of agitation present (Boland et al. 2000; Meagher 2001). If problems persist, subsequent doses can be doubled and given 30 or more minutes apart (Boland et al. 2000; Wise and Trzepacz 1996). Once calm is established, the total dose of haloperidol used over the past 24 hours should be added up and then divided into regularly scheduled doses (Boland et al. 2000). Cardiac monitoring is necessary to avoid the risk of developing excess Q-T prolongation and torsades de pointes (Hunt and Stern 1995; Wilt et al. 1993).

The combination of neuroleptics and benzodiazepines is an excellent alternative when patients fail to respond to neuroleptics alone (Tesar 1993). This combination also reduces the total dose of neuroleptic required to obtain control, possibly lowering the risk of unwanted side effects. Lorazepam usually is chosen because it does not require P450 metabolism, does not produce active metabolites, and is well absorbed by various routes (Meagher 2001). Doses of 0.5–2 mg are normally used and can be given concurrently with haloperidol (Wise and Trzepacz 1996). The use of benzodiazepines alone is not recommended because they can actually worsen mental status (Wise and Trzepacz 1996).

Posttransplant Period

Both survival rates and various measures of function have improved dramatically for transplant recipients. Initially, transplantation is met with a sense of relief and renewed expectations on the part of both the patient and his or her support systems; however, they may fail to view the transplant for what it actually is— an ongoing process that will continue to affect almost every aspect of the patient's life. Living with transplantation requires multiple medications, a protracted recovery period, and the possibility of organ failure. In addition, patients must process the fact that a foreign organ has been placed in their bodies—a concept that may carry a heavy psychological burden. Stability following transplantation can be upset by acute or chronic tissue rejection in addition to numerous psychosocial stresses unique to the posttransplant period. Although transplantation offers life to individuals with end-stage organ failure, impaired functional ability, uncertainty, and psychiatric illness may mark their future.

Psychological Issues

Studies have suggested that the prevalence of depression and anxiety disorders in posttransplant patients is consistent with the prevalence in patients with medical illnesses (Chacko et al. 1996b; Dew et al. 1996a; Freeman et al. 1988). In addition, suicides following successful transplantation have been reported in the literature (Riether and Mahler 1994). With the highly stressful psychological and physical environments of the transplant situation, posttraumatic stress disorder (PTSD) has been recognized in patients and members of their support systems (Dew et al. 1996a; Stukas et al. 1999).

Depression in the posttransplant patient may be the result of a combination of factors, including medication side effects, chronic pain, complicated postoperative course, episodes of rejection, and psychosocial stresses. As with most medically ill patients, the diagnosis of a depressive disorder in a posttransplant patient may be difficult because of the multiple somatic symptoms associated with the posttransplant period. The focus should be on the cognitive and affective components along with somatic complaints that appear to be out of proportion to the patient's current physical condition (Cavenaugh et al. 1983). Collateral data and knowledge of the patient's psychiatric history often assist in the diagnostic process. Depression should not be considered a normal response to the transplant process or a condition that will improve without intervention.

The pharmacological treatment of depression in the posttransplant patient must be approached with careful consideration of medication interactions, the compromised physiological status of the patient, and target symptoms to be treated. Drug interactions between psychopharmacological agents and immunomodulators warrant special attention. Because the cytochrome P450 3A4 enzymes metabolize cyclosporine and tacrolimus, inhibitors of these enzymes can lead to increased levels of immunosuppressants (Olyaci et al. 1998; Vella and Sayegh 1998). Because of the continued risk for delirium in the posttransplant period, medications with significant anticholinergic load or sedative qualities should be used with caution.

With lack of significant cardiovascular, renal, or hepatic toxicity, the SSRIs can be considered first-line treatment. Their ability to treat various anxiety disorders also serves to make them attractive as medication choices in the posttransplant patient. The combined use of fluoxetine and cyclosporine appears to be well tolerated without evidence of increased levels of cyclosporine (Strouse et al. 1996a). Sertraline and paroxetine appear to cause only marginal increases or decreases in cyclosporine concentration (Markowitz et al. 1998). Of the SSRIs, sertraline and citalopram have limited interaction with the cytochrome P450 enzymes (DeVane 1998). Paroxetine is a potent inhibitor of the cytochrome P450 2D6 enzymes, and fluvoxamine strongly inhibits cytochrome P450 3A4, 2C19, and 1A2 enzymes.

Bupropion is generally well tolerated in the medically ill patient, has no significant cardiovascular effects, and has minimal interaction with the cytochrome P450 enzymes (Golden et al. 2001).The lack of sexual side effects of bupropion makes it an attractive alternative to the SSRIs for the posttransplant patient wishing to resume sexual relations. With the possibility of the development of central nervous system lesions and masses in the posttransplant period, the potential seizure risk from the use of bupropion must be considered.

Because of mirtazapine's sedative qualities, its use in the

early posttransplant period may contribute to the development of encephalopathy. Long-term use of mirtazapine has been associated with weight gain, hyperlipidemia, neutropenia, and rare agranulocytosis (R. Davis and Wilde 1996). These conditions can place the posttransplant patient at increased risk for acute and chronic medical conditions; however, careful monitoring of lipid, glucose, weight, and blood cell parameters should allow the safe use of mirtazapine.

Nefazodone, a strong inhibitor of the cytochrome P450 3A4 enzymes, can be used in the treatment of depression with careful monitoring of the levels of various immunosuppressants. Venlafaxine has minimal protein-binding properties and no clinically significant interactions with the various immunosuppressants. The sustained-release formulation of venlafaxine allows once-a-day dosing.

Desipramine and nortriptyline have been used to treat depression in cardiac transplant patients without significant side effects or organ damage; however, with the newer agents that are available, the use of tricyclic antidepressants is not considered first-line management in posttransplant patients (Kay et al. 1991).

There are case reports of posttransplant patients taking methylphenidate to treat cognitive slowing, dysphoric mood, social withdrawal, apathy, and amotivational behavior (Plutchik et al. 1998). Initial doses tend to be 5 mg in the morning with eventual target doses of 10–20 mg/day (Plutchik et al. 1998). The use of pemoline should be avoided in the transplant patient because of its association with hepatic toxicity and failure. Modafinil, which has a unique mechanism of action differing from that of methylphenidate, is an alternative for the augmentation of antidepressants (Menza et al. 2000); however, modafinil may induce the cytochrome P450 3A4 enzymes, leading to potential decreases in cyclosporine and tacrolimus levels.

With the increase in the use of complementary and alternative medicine, posttransplant patients need to be carefully screened for the use of herbal and nonherbal supplements in the self-treatment of depression and anxiety. The use of St. John's wort (*Hypericum perforatum*) has been associated with decreased cyclosporine levels (I. Mai et al. 2000). This is most likely caused by the induction of the cytochrome P450 3A4 enzymes.

Anxiety disorders are a common psychiatric occurrence in the posttransplant period. Adjustment disorders with anxious mood have an incidence of approximately 5%–15% in posttransplant patients (Dew et al. 1996a; Freeman et al. 1988). Generalized anxiety disorder appears to be much less common (Fukunishi 1993). Specific situations unique to the posttransplant period that may lead to increased anxiety include discharge from the hospital, acute and chronic tissue rejection, infection, and financial burdens.

The development of PTSD in heart transplant patients and their caregivers recently has been examined (Dew et al. 1996a; Stukas et al. 1999). In their study, Stukas et al. (1999) found that 10.5% of the transplant patients and 7.7% of their caregivers met full criteria for PTSD. The caregivers were more likely to experience rapid onset of symptoms as compared with the transplant patients. Both the patients and the caregivers considered learning of the need for transplant and the variable waiting period to be significant traumatic events (Stukas et al. 1999). Having histories of psychiatric illness, being female or of younger ages, and lacking a cohesive family structure predisposed study participants to the development of PTSD (Stukas et al. 1999).

In general, anxiety symptoms can be treated based on the recommendations outlined in the pretransplant section with consideration of drug-drug interactions unique to the posttransplant period. Buspirone may have a role in decreasing alcohol consumption, making it a possible anxiolytic choice in the posttransplant alcoholic patient (Tollefson et al. 1999).

Careful attention to the possibility of substance abuse and dependence is critical in the posttransplant period. Although recidivism tends to be fairly low in the first year after transplant, the incidence increases significantly at 2- to 3-year follow-up (Gerhardt et al. 1998). Coffman et al. (1997) suggested that alcohol relapse is correlated with low quality-of-life measures following liver transplantation. Various studies found that alcohol consumption is probably underreported in the posttransplant population (Berlakovich et al. 1999). A recent study by DiMartini et al. (2001) showed that clinical interviews by a transplant psychiatrist were more likely than biological markers to detect alcohol use in the posttransplant period.

Neurocognitive Recovery

Neurocognitive status following transplantation has implications in the areas of psychological, social, and occupational functioning. In addition, compliance with posttransplant routines may be compromised by neurocognitive declines in the areas of memory and executive function. Cognitive difficulties, especially those associated with the development of pretransplant encephalopathy, tend to improve or resolve after transplantation (Powell et al. 1999). Arria et al. (1991) found that alcoholic cirrhotic patients who had undergone liver transplantation had improved visuopractic, psychomotor, and abstracting abilities at 1-year follow-up; however, memory was not significantly improved. B. Jones et al. (1992) found that a cohort of heart transplant patients showed improvement in short-term memory, psychomotor speed, planning ability, visual memory, and mental calculations 4 months after transplantation.

It is not clear whether cognitive difficulties in the posttransplant period are caused by irreversible neurological damage before transplantation, new factors present in the posttransplant period, or a combination. It is often difficult to determine patient baseline cognitive functioning prior to the development of end-stage organ failure. Further research in this area is needed, but the general trend appears to be improvement in neurocognitive functions posttransplant.

Quality of Life

With the increasing rates of solid organ transplantation and improved survival rates, much research has been conducted in the area of quality of life following transplantation. The body of work has broad implications for issues such as health care costs, use of limited resources, termination of medical treatment, and risk-benefit ratios (Joralemon and Fujinaga 1996).

Quality-of-life studies in the transplant literature are numerous, varied, and difficult to interpret. Multiple instruments have been used to measure quality of life, hindering comparability. Sample sizes vary, and the inclusion and types of comparison groups are not consistent. In addition, the definitions of the domains and their variables that are examined in the quality-of-life studies vary. Methodological formats vary from medical record reviews and case reports to systematic evaluation at various stages of the treatment process. Finally, the length of time from transplant to inclusion in a study varies.

Domains that have been studied include overall physical functioning, psychological and cognitive areas, and social functioning. Variables within physical functioning include mobility/ambulation, pain, fatigue/energy level, sleep, and physical activity/endurance. Examination of psychological functioning tends to focus on depression, anxiety, and self-esteem/self-image. Cognitive functioning examines memory impairment, executive functions, attention, and concentration. The social domain often includes employment status, marital status, sexual functioning, leisure activities, and family functioning. In the domain of physical functioning, most studies regardless of type of organ transplanted have reported posttransplant improvement. The most significant improvement has been found in the heart, lung, lung/heart, and pancreas groups (Dew et al. 2000a). Dew et al. (2000a) found less robust improvement in the liver and kidney transplant groups. Variables studied included activities of daily living, functional constraints, perceived overall health, and satisfaction with health status.

Psychological functioning following transplantation is generally marked by improvement from pretransplant status. However, most studies indicate that when compared with physical functioning, psychological functioning shows less of an improvement. Pretransplant psychological functioning does appear to have a significant effect on posttransplant psychological status (Dew et al. 1997; Grady et al. 1999). This finding strengthens the need to identify and appropriately treat psychological distress in the pretransplant period. Studies have found that depression is relatively common in posttransplant patients (Commander et al. 1992; Paris et al. 1994).

Employment status is often considered a major variable for

the social domain of quality-of-life studies. The rates of employment tend to be higher after transplantation and compared with control groups; however, studies found wide variability between and within transplant groups (Botsford 1992; Gorlen et al. 1993). Sexual functioning tends to improve following transplantation and is often associated with increased satisfaction in marital or long-term relationships (Frazier et al. 1995; Mulligan et al. 1991). However, posttransplant patients are less satisfied with sexual relationships than are control subjects who did not receive transplants. Heart transplant patients appear to have the most difficulty with sexual functioning or libido following transplantation (McAleer et al. 1985; Shapiro and Kornfeld 1989). In all transplant groups, social interest and family relationships tend to show at least mild improvement from pretransplant measures.

Quality-of-life studies examine overall satisfaction less often than specific domains. It is clear that perceived global quality of life improves after transplant in most studies. This trend suggests that the domains that usually are studied in isolation may not fully evaluate a patient's quality of life (Powell et al. 1999). In addition, most studies examine global quality of life by comparing posttransplant patients with medically ill control subjects instead of healthy control subjects.

Conclusion

Patients are evaluated for transplantation while they are coping with declining health and increasing dependence on others. Not appearing at their best, some patients also have concurrent psychiatric or substance abuse disorders complicating the task of evaluation. Relief that comes from being placed on the waiting list is tempered by the question of surviving until a donor organ becomes available. In this uncertain period, depression and anxiety are common. After the donor organ is sutured in, new hurdles appear, including a prolonged recovery period and the effects of immunosuppression. Given the difficulties that may arise at each step in the transplant process, psychiatric input at each step can help to reach the goal of physical and psychological recovery from end-stage organ disease.

References

Abosh D, Rosser B, Kaita K, et al: Outcomes following liver transplantation for patients with alcohol- versus nonalcohol-induced liver disease. Can J Gastroenterol 14:851–855, 2000

Abramowicz M: Some drugs that cause psychiatric symptoms. Med Lett Drugs Ther 40:21–24, 1998

Adams DH, Ponsford S, Gunson B, et al: Neurological complications following liver transplantation. Lancet 1:949–951, 1987

American Psychiatric Association: Diagnostic and Statistical Manual of Mental Disorders, 4th Edition, Text Revision. Washington, DC, American Psychiatric Association, 2000

Arria A, Tarter R, Starzl T, et al: Improvement in cognitive functioning of alcoholics following orthotopic liver transplantation. Alcohol Clin Exp Res 15:956–962, 1991

Aulisio MP, Arnold RM: Exclusionary criteria and suicidal behavior: comment on "should a patient who attempted suicide receive a liver transplant?" Journal of Clinical Ethics 7:277–283, 1996

Bakti G, Fisch H, Karaganis G, et al: Mechanism of the sedative response of cirrhotics to benzodiazepines: model experiments with triazolam. Hepatology 7:629–638, 1987

Barbhaiya R, Brady M, Shukla U, et al: Steady state pharmacokinetics of nefazodone in subjects with normal and impaired renal function. Eur J Clin Pharmacol 49:229–235, 1995

Beautrais AL: Suicides and serious suicide attempts: two populations or one? Psychol Med 31:837–845, 2001

Beliles KE: Alternate routes of administration of psychotropic agents, in Psychiatric Care of the Medical Patient, 2nd Edition. Edited by Stoudemire A, Fogel BS, Greenberg DB. New York, Oxford University Press, 2000, pp 395–405

Beliles K, Stoudemire A: Psychopharmacologic treatment of depression in the medically ill. Psychosomatics 39:S2–S19, 1998

Benning C, Smith A: Psychosocial needs of family members of liver transplant patients. Clinical Nurse Specialists 5:280–288, 1994

Beresford TP, Turcotte JG, Merion R, et al: A rational approach to liver transplantation for the alcoholic patient. Psychosomatics 31:241–253, 1990

Berlakovich G, Windhager T, Freundorfer E, et al: Carbohydrate deficient transferrin for detection of alcohol relapse after orthotopic liver transplantation for alcoholic cirrhosis. Transplantation 67:1231–1235, 1999

Boland RJ, Goldstein MG, Haltzman SD: Psychiatric management of behavioral syndromes in intensive care units, in Psychiatric Care of the Medical Patient, 2nd Edition. Edited by Stoudemire A, Fogel BS, Greenberg DB. New York, Oxford University Press, 2000, pp 299–314

Boston Collaborative Drug Surveillance Program: Acute adverse reaction to prednisone in relation to dosage. Clin Pharmacother 13:694–697, 1972

Botsford A: Review of literature on heart transplant recipients' return to work: predictors and outcomes. Transplantation 53:1038–1040, 1992

Brennan AF, Davis MH, Bucholz DJ, et al: Predictors of quality of life following cardiac transplantation. Psychosomatics 28:566–571, 1987

Bronster DJ, Gurkhan A, Buchsbaum MS, et al: Tacrolimus-associated mutism after orthotopic liver transplantation. Transplantation 70:79–982, 2000

Brown T, Stoudemire A: Antidepressants, in Psychiatric Side Effects of Prescription and Over-the-Counter Medications. Washington, DC, American Psychiatric Press, 1998, pp 53–82

Brown T, Stoudemire A, Fogel B, et al: Psychopharmacology in the medical patient, in Psychiatric Care of the Medical Patient, 2nd Edition. Edited by Stoudemire A, Fogel BS, Greenberg DB. New York, Oxford University Press, 2000, pp 329–372

Bunzel B, Laederach-Hoffman K: Solid organ transplantation: are there predictors for posttransplant noncompliance? A literature overview. Transplantation 70:711–716, 2000

Buse S, Pieper B: Impact of cardiac transplantation on the spouse's life. Heart Lung 19:641–648, 1990

Cadranel J, El Younsi M, Pidoux B, et al: Flumazenil therapy for hepatic encephalopathy in cirrhotic patients: a double-blind pragmatic randomized, placebo study. Eur J Gastroenterol Hepatol 7:325–329, 1995

Campbell DA, Punch JD: Monitoring for alcohol use relapse after liver transplantation for alcoholic liver disease. Liver Transpl Surg 3:300–303, 1997

Cavenaugh S, Clark D, Gibbons R: Diagnosing depression in the hospitalized medically ill. Psychosomatics 24:809–815, 1983

Chacko RC, Harper RG, Gotto J, et al: Psychiatric interview and psychometric predictors of cardiac transplant survival. Am J Psychiatry 153:1607–1612, 1996a

Chacko RC, Harper RG, Kunig M, et al: Relationship of psychiatric morbidity and psychosocial factors in organ transplant candidates. Psychosomatics 37:100–107, 1996b

Clemmensen J, Larsen F, Kondrup J, et al: Cerebral herniation in patients with acute liver failure is correlated with arterial ammonia concentration. Hepatology 29:648–653, 1999

Coffman KL, Crone CC: Transplantation in patients with histories of psychotic disorder (abstract). Psychosomatics 40:139, 1999

Coffman K, Hoffman A, Sher L, et al: Treatment of postoperative alcoholic liver transplant recipient with other addictions. Liver Transpl Surg 3:322–327, 1997

Collins E, White-Williams C, Jalowiec A: Impact of the heart transplant waiting process on spouses. J Heart Lung Transplant 15:623–630, 1996

Commander M, Neuberger J, Dean C: Psychiatric and social consequences of liver transplantation. Transplantation 53:1038–1040, 1992

Craven J: Psychiatric aspects of organ transplantation. Med Clin North Am 37:657–662, 1989

Craven JL, Toronto Lung Transplant Group: Postoperative organic mental syndromes in lung transplant recipients. Journal of Heart Transplantation 9(2):129–132, 1990

Crone CC, Wise TN: Psychiatric aspects of organ transplantation, III: postoperative issues. Critical Care Nurse 19:28–38, 1999a

Crone CC, Wise TN: Psychiatric aspects of transplantation, I: evaluation and selection of candidates. Critical Care Nurse 19:79–87, 1999b

Culledge D, Buszta C, Montague DK: Psychosocial aspects of renal transplantation. Urol Clin North Am 10:327–335, 1983

Cunningham L, Borison R, Carman J, et al: A comparison of venlafaxine, trazodone, and placebo in major depression. J Clin Psychopharmacol 14:99–106, 1994

Dalhoff K, Almdal T, Bjerrum K, et al: Pharmacokinetics of paroxetine in patients with cirrhosis. Eur J Clin Pharmacol 41:351–354, 1991

Davis GL: Current therapy for chronic hepatitis C. Gastroenterology 118:S104–S114, 2000

Davis R, Wilde M: Mirtazapine: a review of its pharmacology and therapeutic potential in the management of major depression. CNS Drugs 5:389–402, 1996

de Boer T: The pharmacological profile of mirtazapine. J Clin Psychiatry 57 (suppl 4):19–25, 1996

De Geest S, Abraham I, Moons P, et al: Late acute rejection and subclinical noncompliance with cyclosporine therapy in heart transplant recipients. J Heart Lung Transplant 17:854–863, 1998 de Groen P, Craven J: Organic brain syndromes in transplant patients, in Psychiatric Aspects of Organ Transplantation. Edited by Craven J, Rodin GM. New York, Oxford University Press, 1992, pp 67–88

de Groen PC, Aksamit AJ, Rakela J, et al: Central nervous system toxicity after liver transplantation: the role if cyclosporine and cholesterol. N Engl J Med 317:861–866, 1987

de Groen PC, Weisner RH, Krom RA: Advanced liver failure predisposes to cyclosporine-induced central nervous system symptoms after liver transplantation. Transplant Proc 21 (1 pt 1):2456, 1989

DeMarinis N, Rynn M, Rickels K, et al: Prior benzodiazepine use and buspirone response in the treatment of generalized anxiety disorder. J Clin Psychiatry 61:91–94, 2000

Demolis J, Angebaud P, Grange J, et al: Influence of liver cirrhosis on sertraline pharmacokinetics. Br J Clin Pharmacol 42:394–397, 1996

Deshields T, McDonough E, Mannen R, et al: Psychological and cognitive status before and after heart transplantation. Gen Hosp Psychiatry 18:62S–69S, 1996

DeVane C: Drug therapy for anxiety and insomnia, in Fundamentals of Monitoring Psychoactive Drug Therapy. Edited by DeVane C. Baltimore, MD, Williams & Wilkins, 1990, pp 191–238

DeVane CL: Principles of pharmacokinetics and pharmacodynamics, in The American Psychiatric Press Textbook of Psychopharmacology, 2nd Edition. Edited by Schatzberg AF, Nemeroff CB. Washington, DC, American Psychiatric Press, 1998, pp 155–169

Dew MA, Kormos R: Early post-transplant medical compliance and mental health predict physical morbidity and mortality one to three years after heart transplantation. J Heart Lung Transplant 18:549–562, 1999

Dew M, Roth L, Schulberg H, et al: Prevalence and predictors of depression and anxiety-related disorders during the year after heart transplant. Gen Hosp Psychiatry 18:48S–61S, 1996a

Dew MA, Roth LH, Thompson ME, et al: Medical compliance and its predictors in the first year after heart transplantation. J Heart Lung Transplant 15:631–645, 1996b

Dew M, Switzer G, Gocoolea J, et al: Does transplantation produce quality of life benefits? Transplantation 64:1261–1273, 1997

Dew M, Goycoolea J, Switzer G, et al: Quality of life in organ transplantation: effects on adult recipients and their families, in The Transplant Patient. Edited by Trzepacz P, DiMartini A. Cambridge, UK, Cambridge University Press, 2000a, pp 67–145

Dew MA, Switzer GE, DiMartini AF, et al: Psychosocial assessments and outcomes in organ transplantation. Progress in Transplantation 10:239–261, 2000b

DiMartini A, Trzepacz P: Psychopharmacologic issues in organ transplantation, in Cutting Edge Medicine and Liaison Psychiatry. Edited by Matsushita M, Fukunishi I. Amsterdam, Elsevier, 1999, pp 111–119

DiMartini AF, Trzepacz PT: Alcoholism and organ transplantation, in The Transplant Patient: Biological, Psychiatric, and Ethical Issues in Organ Transplantation. Edited by Trzepacz P, DiMartini A. Cambridge, UK, Cambridge University Press, 2000, pp 214–238

DiMartini AF, Twillman R: Organ transplantation and paranoid schizophrenia. Psychosomatics 35:159–161, 1994

DiMartini A, Magill J, Fitzgerald MG, et al: Use of a high-risk alcohol relapse scale in evaluating liver transplant candidates. Alcohol Clin Exp Res 24:1198–1201, 2000

DiMartini A, Day N, Dew M, et al: Alcohol use following liver transplantation: a comparison of follow-up methods. Psychosomatics 42:55–62, 2001

Dobbels F, Put C, Vanhaecke J: Personality disorders: a challenge for transplantation. Progress in Transplantation 10:226–232, 2000

Douglas S, Blixen C, Bartucci MR: Relationship between pre-transplant noncompliance and posttransplant outcomes in renal transplant recipients. J Transpl Coord 6:53–58, 1996

Eidelman BH, Abu-Elmagd K, Wilson J, et al: Neurologic complications of FK 506. Transplant Proc 23:3175–3178, 1991

Everhart JE, Beresford TP: Liver transplantation for alcoholic liver disease: a survey of transplantation programs in the United States. Liver Transpl Surg 3:220–226, 1997

Everson G, Bharadhwaj G, House R, et al: Long-term follow up of patients with alcoholic liver disease who underwent hepatic transplantation. Liver Transpl Surg 3:263–274, 1997

Fish DN: Treatment of delirium in the critically ill patient. Clinical Pharmacy 10:456–466, 1991

Fontana RJ, Quallich LG: Acute liver failure. Gastroenterology 17:291–298, 2001

Forster J, Bartholome WG, Delcore R: Should a patient who attempted suicide receive a liver transplant? J Clin Ethics 7:257–267, 1996

Frazier P, Davis-Ali S, Dahl K: Stressors, social support, and adjustment in kidney transplant patients and their spouses. Soc Work Health Care 21:93–108, 1995

Freeman AM, Folks DG, Sokol RS: Cardiac transplantation: clinical correlates of psychiatric outcome. Psychosomatics 29:47–54, 1988

Fricchione GL: Psychiatric aspects of renal transplantation. Aust N Z J Psychiatry 23:407–417, 1989

Fukunishi I: Anxiety associated with kidney transplantation. Psychopathology 26:24–28, 1993

Furmaga KM, DeLeon OA, Sinha SB, et al: Psychosis in medical conditions: response to risperidone. Gen Hosp Psychiatry 19:223–228, 1997

Garner S, Eldridge F, Wagner P, et al: Buspirone, an anxiolytic drug that stimulates respiration. Am Rev Respir Dis 139:946–950, 1989

Gaston RS, Hudson SL, Ward M, et al: Late renal allograft loss: noncompliance masquerading as chronic rejection. Transplant Proc 31 (suppl 4A):21S–23S, 1999

Gerhardt TC, Goldstein RM, Urschel HC, et al: Alcohol use following liver transplantation for alcoholic cirrhosis. Transplantation 62:1060–1063, 1998

Goldberg RJ, Posner DA: Anxiety in the medically ill, in Psychiatric Care of the Medical Patient, 2nd Edition. Edited by Stoudemire A, Fogel BS, Greenberg DB. New York, Oxford University Press, 2000, pp 165–180

Golden R, Dawkins K, Nicholas L, et al: Trazodone, nefazodone, bupropion, and mirtazapine, in Essentials of Clinical Psychopharmacology. Edited by Schatzberg A, Nemeroff C. Washington, DC, American Psychiatric Publishing, 2001, pp 55–74

Gordon MJV, White R, Matas AJ, et al: Renal transplantation in patients with a history of heroin abuse. Transplantation 42:556–557, 1986

Gorlen T, Ekeberg O, Abdelnoor M, et al: Quality of life after kidney transplantation: a 10–22 year follow-up. Scand J Urol Nephrol 27:89–92, 1993

Grady K, Jalowiec A, White-Williams C: Predictors of quality of life in patients at one year after heart transplantation. J Heart Lung Transplant 18:202–210, 1999

Greene D, Barbhaiya R: Clinical pharmacokinetics of nefazodone. Clin Pharmacokinet 33:260–275, 1997

Greenstein S, Siegal B: Compliance and noncompliance in patients with a functioning renal transplant: a multicenter study. Transplantation 66:1718–1726, 1998

Greiner C: Evaluation of acetaminophen overdosage patients for liver transplantation. Paper presented at the First Working Conference on the Psychiatric, Psychosocial, and Ethical Aspects of Organ Transplantation, Toronto, Ontario, September 1990

Gross C, Malinchoc M, Kim W, et al: Quality of life before and after liver transplantation for cholestatic liver disease. Hepatology 29:356–364, 1999

Gry K, Meier R, Haussler J, et al: Evaluation of the efficacy and safety of flumazenil in the treatment of portal systemic encephalopathy: a double blind, randomized, placebo controlled multicentre study. Gut 39:319–324, 1996

Guarino M, Stracciari A, Pazzaglia P, et al: Neurological complications of liver transplantation. J Neurol 243:137–142, 1996

Hall RC, Popkin MK, Stickney SK, et al: Presentation of the steroid psychoses. J Nerv Ment Dis 167:229–236, 1979

Hauben M: Cyclosporine neurotoxicity. Pharmacotherapy 16:576–583, 1996

Haynes R, McKibbon K, Kanani R: Systematic review of randomised trials of interventions to assist patients to follow prescriptions for medications. Lancet 348:383–386, 1996

Hazell A, Butterworth R: Hepatic encephalopathy: an update of pathophysiologic mechanisms. Proc Soc Exp Biol Med 222:99–112, 1999

Hickey M, Leske J: Needs of families of critically ill patients: state of the science and future direction. Critical Care Nursing Clinics of North America 4:645–649, 1992

Hoofnagle JH, Kresina T, Fuller RK, et al: Liver transplantation for alcoholic liver disease: executive statement and recommendations—summary of a National Institutes of Health Workshop held December 6–7, 1996, Bethesda, Maryland. Liver Transpl Surg 3:347–350, 1997

House RM, Thompson TL: Psychiatric aspects of organ transplantation. JAMA 260:535–539, 1988

House R, Dubovsky S, Penn I: Psychiatric aspects of hepatic transplantation. Transplantation 36:146–150, 1983

Hunt N, Stern TA: The association between intravenous haloperidol and torsades de pointes: three cases and a literature review. Psychosomatics 36:541–549, 1995

Jalowiec A, Grady K, White-Williams C: Stressors in patients awaiting a heart transplant. Behav Med 19:145–154, 1994

Jones B, Taylor F, Downs K, et al: Long-term follow-up of the emotional adjustment of patients after heart transplantation, in Quality of Life After Open Heart Surgery. Edited by Walter PJ. Dordrecht, Netherlands, Kluwer Academic Publishers, 1992, pp 427–437

Jones E, Weissenborn K: Neurology and the liver. J Neurol Neurosurg Psychiatry 63:279–293, 1997

Joralemon D, Fujinaga K: Studying the quality of life after organ transplantation: research problems and solutions. Soc Sci Med 44:1259–1269, 1996

Joseph H, Stancliff S, Langrod J: Methadone maintenance treatment (MMT): a review of historical and clinical issues. Mt Sinai J Med 67:347–364, 2000

Kay J, Bienenfeld D, Slomowitz M, et al: Use of tricyclic antidepressants in recipients of heart transplants. Psychosomatics 32:165–170, 1991

Kershner P, Wang-Cheng R: Psychiatric side effects of steroid therapy. Psychosomatics 30:135–139, 1989

Kiev A, Masco H, Wenger T, et al: The cardiovascular effects of bupropion and nortriptyline in depressed outpatients. Ann Clin Psychiatry 6:107–115, 1994

Kim HF, Kunik ME, Molinari VA, et al: Functional impairment in COPD patients: the impact of anxiety and depression. Psychosomatics 41:465–471, 2000

Koch M, Banys P: Liver transplantation and opioid dependence. JAMA 285:1056–1058, 2001

Kuhn W, Brennan A, Lacefield P, et al: Psychiatric distress during stages of the heart transplant protocol. Heart Transplant 9:25–29, 1990

Kumar S, Stauber RE, Gavaler JS, et al: Orthotopic liver transplantation for alcoholic liver disease. Hepatology 11:159–164, 1990

Levenson JL, Dwight M: Cardiology, in Psychiatric Care of the Medical Patient, 2nd Edition. Edited by Stoudemire A, Fogel BS, Greenberg DB. New York, Oxford University Press, 2000, pp 717–731

Levenson J, Olbrisch M: Shortage of donor organs and long waits: new sources of stress for transplant patients. Psychosomatics 28:399–406, 1987

Levenson JL, Olbrisch ME: A comparative survey of process, criteria, and outcomes in heart, liver, and kidney transplantation. Psychosomatics 34:314–323, 1993

Levenson JL, Olbrisch ME: Psychosocial screening and selection of candidates for organ transplantation, in The Transplant Patient: Biological, Psychiatric, and Ethical Issues in Organ Transplantation. Edited by Trzepacz P, DiMartini A. Cambridge, UK, Cambridge University Press, 2000, pp 21–41

Levy NB: Psychopharmacology in patients with renal failure. Int J Psychiatry Med 20:325–334, 1990

Lewis DA, Smith RE: Steroid-induced psychiatric syndromes. J Affect Disord 5:319–322, 1983

Liptzkin B: Clinical diagnosis and management of delirium, in Psychiatric Care of the Medical Patient, 2nd Edition. Edited by Stoudemire A, Fogel BS, Greenberg DB. New York, Oxford University Press, 2000, pp 581–596

Litaker D, Locala J, Franco K, et al: Preoperative risk factors for postoperative delirium. Gen Hosp Psychiatry 23:84–89, 2001

Mai F: Psychiatric aspects of heart transplantation. Br J Psychiatry 163:285–292, 1993

Mai I, Kruger H, Budde K, et al: Hazardous pharmacokinetic interaction of Saint John's wort (Hypericum perforatum) with the immunosuppressant cyclosporin. Int J Clin Pharmacol Ther 38:500–502, 2000

Markowitz J, Gill H, Hunt N, et al: Lack of antidepressant-cyclosporine pharmacokinetic interactions (letter). J Clin Psychopharmacol 18:91–93, 1998

Mayou RA, Gill D, Thompson DR, et al: Depression and anxiety as predictors of outcome after myocardial infarction. Psychosom Med 62:212–219, 2000

McAleer M, Copeland J, Fuller J, et al: Psychological aspects of heart transplantation. Heart Transplant 4:232–233, 1985

McDaniel JS, Brown FW, Cole SA: Assessment of depression and grief reactions in the medically ill, in Psychiatric Care of the Medical Patient, 2nd Edition. Edited by Stoudemire A, Fogel BS, Greenberg DB. New York, Oxford University Press, 2000, pp 149–164

McDiarmid SV, Busuttil RW, Ascher NL, et al: FK506 (tacrolimus) compared with cyclosporine for primary immunosuppression after pediatric liver transplantation: results from the U.S. multicenter trial. Transplantation 59:530–536, 1995

McGuire BE, Basten CJ, Ryan CJ, et al: Intensive care unit syndrome: a dangerous misnomer. Arch Intern Med 7:906–909, 2000

Meagher DJ: Delirium: optimising management. BMJ 322:144–149, 2001

Menza MA, Murray GB, Holmes VF, et al: Decreased extrapyramidal symptoms with intravenous haloperidol. J Clin Psychiatry 48:278–280, 1987

Menza M, Kaufman K, Castellanos A: Modafinil augmentation of antidepressant treatment in depression. J Clin Psychiatry 61:378–381, 2000

Michalak A, Butterworth R: Selective loss of binding sites for the glutamate receptor ligands [3H] kainate and (S)-[3H] 5-fluorowillardine in the brains of rats with acute liver failure. Hepatology 25:631–635, 1997

Miller LW: Cyclosporine-associated neurotoxicity: the need for a better guide for immunosuppressive therapy. Circulation 94:1209–1211, 1996

Montgomery S: Safety of mirtazapine: a review. Int Clin Psychopharmacol 10 (suppl 4):37–45, 1995

Mori DL, Gallagher P, Milne J: The Structured Interview for Renal Transplantation—SIRT. Psychosomatics 41:393–406, 2000

Moss AH, Siegler M: Should alcoholics compete equally for liver transplantation? JAMA 265:1295–1298, 1991

Mulligan T, Sheehan H, Hanrahan J: Sexual function after heart transplantation. J Heart Lung Transplant 10:125–128, 1991

National organ transplant waiting list tops 75,000. UNOS Update, April 2001

Nelson MK, Presberg BA, Olbrisch ME, et al: Behavioral contingency contracting to reduce substance abuse and other high-risk health behaviors in organ transplant patients. J Transpl Coord 5:35–40, 1995

Ninan P, Cole J, Yonkers K: Nonbenzodiazepine anxiolytics, in The American Psychiatric Press Textbook of Psychopharmacology, 2nd Edition. Edited by Schatzberg AF, Nemeroff CB. Washington, DC, American Psychiatric Press, 1998, pp 287–299

Nolan M, Cupples S, Brown M, et al: Perceived stress and coping strategies among families of cardiac transplant candidates during the organ waiting period. Heart Lung 21:540–547, 1992

Norenberg M, Huo Z, Neary J, et al: The glial glutamate transporter in hyperammonemia and hepatic encephalopathy: relation to energy metabolism and glutamatergic neurotransmission. Glia 21:124–133, 1997

Olbrisch ME, Levenson JL: Psychosocial assessment of organ transplant candidates: current status of methodological and philosophical issues. Psychosomatics 36:236–243, 1995

Olbrisch ME, Levenson JL, Hamer R: The PACT: a rating scale for the study of clinical decision making in psychosocial screening of organ transplant candidates. Clin Transplant 3:164–169, 1989

Olyaci A, deMattos A, Norman D, et al: Interactions between tacrolimus and nefazodone in a stable renal transplant recipient. Pharmacotherapy 18:1356–1359, 1998

Pageaux GP, Michel J, Coste V, et al: Alcoholic cirrhosis is a good indication for liver transplantation, even for cases of recidivism. Gut 45:421–426, 1999

Papp L, Sinha S, Martinez J, et al: Low dose venlafaxine treatment in panic disorder. Psychopharmacol Bull 34:207–210, 1998

Paris W, Muchmore J, Pribil A, et al: Study of the relative incidences of psychosocial factors before and after heart transplantation and the influence of posttransplantation psychosocial factors on heart transplantation outcome. J Heart Lung Transplant 13:424–432, 1994

Pereira SP, Williams R: Liver transplantation for alcoholic liver disease at King's College Hospital: survival and quality of life. Liver Transpl Surg 3:245–250, 1997

Phipps L: Psychiatric aspects of heart transplantation. Can J Psychiatry 36:297–307, 1991

Plutchik L, Snyder S, Drooker M, et al: Methylphenidate in post liver transplant patients. Psychosomatics 39:118–123, 1998

Pohl R, Wolkow R, Clary C: Sertraline in the treatment of panic disorder: a double-blind multicentered trial. Am J Psychiatry 155:1189–1895, 1998

Powell E, Pender M, Chalk J, et al: Improvement in chronic hepatocerebral degeneration following liver transplantation. Gastroenterology 98:1079–1082, 1999

Quero J, Schalm S: Subclinical hepatic encephalopathy. Semin Liver Dis 16:321–328, 1996

Rabkin JM, Oroloff SL, Corless CL, et al: Association of fungal infection and increased mortality in liver transplant recipients. Am J Surg 179:426–430, 2000

Rickels K, Downing R, Schweizer E, et al: Antidepressants for the treatment of generalized anxiety disorder. Arch Gen Psychiatry 50:884–890, 1993

Riether A, Mahler E: Suicide in liver transplant patients. Psychosomatics 35:574–578, 1994

Rodin G, Abbey S: Kidney transplantation, in Psychiatric Aspects of Organ Transplantation. Edited by Craven J, Rodin GM. New York, Oxford University Press, 1992, pp 145–163

Roose S, Dalack G, Glassman A, et al: Cardiovascular effects of bupropion in depressed patients with heart disease. Am J Psychiatry 148:512–516, 1991

Rosenblum D, Rosen M, Pine Z, et al: Health status and quality of life following cardiac transplantation. Arch Phys Med Rehabil 74:490–493, 1993

Schenker S, Perkins HS, Sorrell MF: Should patients with end-stage alcoholic liver disease have a new liver? Hepatology 11:314–319, 1990

Selby R, Ramirez CB, Singh R, et al: Brain abscess in organ transplant recipients receiving cyclosporine-based immunosuppression. Arch Surg 132:304–310, 1997

Shapiro P, Kornfeld D: Psychiatric outcome of heart transplantation. Gen Hosp Psychiatry 11:352–357, 1989

Shapiro PA, Williams DL, Foray AT, et al: Psychosocial evaluation and prediction of compliance problems and morbidity after heart transplantation. Transplantation 60(12):1462–1466, 1995

Siegel BR, Greenstein SM: Postrenal transplant compliance from the perspective of African-Americans, Hispanic Americans, and Anglo-Americans. Adv Ren Replace Ther 4:46–54, 1997

Singh N, Bonham A, Fukui M: Immunosuppressive-associated leuko-encephalopathy in organ transplant recipients. Transplantation 69:467–472, 2000

Sipahimalani A, Masand PS: Olanzapine in the treatment of delirium. Psychosomatics 39:422–430, 1998

Smoller J, Pollack M, Otto M, et al: Panic anxiety, dyspnea, respiratory disease. Am J Respir Crit Care Med 154:6–17, 1996

Spiller H, Ramoska E, Krenzelok E: Buproprion overdose: a 3 year multicenter retrospective analysis. Am J Emerg Med 12:43–45, 1994

Stoudemire A: Epidemiology and psychopharmacology of anxiety in medical patients. J Clin Psychiatry 57 (suppl 7):64–72, 1996

Strouse T, Salehmoghaddam S, Spar J: Acute delirium and parkinsonism in a buproprion-treated liver transplant recipient (letter). J Clin Psychiatry 54:489–490, 1993

Strouse T, Fairbanks L, Skotzko C, et al: Fluoxetine and cyclosporine in organ transplantation. Psychosomatics 37:23–30, 1996a

Strouse TB, Wolcott DL, Skotzko CE: Transplantation, in The American Psychiatric Press Textbook of Consultation-Liaison Psychiatry. Edited by Rundell JR, Wise MG. Washington, DC, American Psychiatric Press, 1996b, pp 640–670

Stukas A, Dew M, Switzer G, et al: PTSD in heart transplant recipients and their primary family caregivers. Psychosomatics 40:212–221, 1999

Surman OS: Psychiatric aspects of organ transplantation. Am J Psychiatry 146:972–982, 1989

Surman OS: Psychiatric aspects of liver transplantation. Psychosomatics 35:297–307, 1994

Tarter RE, Switala J: Cognitive assessment in organ transplantation, in The Transplant Patient: Biological, Psychiatric, and Ethical Issues in Organ Transplantation. Edited by Trzepacz P, DiMartini A. Cambridge, UK, Cambridge University Press, 2000, pp 164–186

Tesar GE: The agitated patient, part II: pharmacologic treatment. Hospital and Community Psychiatry 44:627–629, 1993

Tesar GE, Stern TA: Evaluation and treatment of agitation in the intensive care unit. J Intensive Care Med 1:137–148, 1986

Thompson WL: Pulmonary disease, in Psychiatric Care of the Medical Patient, 2nd Edition. Edited by Stoudemire A, Fogel BS, Greenberg DB. New York, Oxford University Press, 2000, pp 757–774

Tollefson G, Rosenbaum J: Selective serotonin reuptake inhibitors, in The American Psychiatric Press Textbook of Psychopharmacology, 2nd Edition. Edited by Schatzberg AF, Nemeroff CB. Washington, DC, American Psychiatric Press, 1998, pp 219–237

Tollefson G, Lancaster S, Montagne-Clouse J: The association of buspirone and its metabolite l-pyrimidinylpiperazine in the remission of co-morbid anxiety with depressive features and alcohol dependency. Psychopharmacol Bull 27:163–170, 1999

Tringali RA, Trzepacz PT, DiMartini A, et al: Assessment and follow-up of alcohol-dependent liver transplantation patients—a clinical cohort. Gen Hosp Psychiatry 18:70S–77S, 1996

Trumper A, Appleby L: Psychiatric morbidity in patients undergoing heart, heart and lung, or lung transplantation. J Psychosom Res 50:103–105, 2001

Trzepacz PT: Pharmacologic issues in organ transplantation, in The Transplant Patient: Biological, Psychiatric, and Ethical Issues in Organ Transplantation. Edited by Trzepacz P, DiMartini A. Cambridge, UK, Cambridge University Press, 2000, pp 187–213

Trzepacz PT, Francis J: Low serum albumin and risk of delirium (letter). Am J Psychiatry 147:675, 1990

Trzepacz PT, Brenner R, Van Thiel DH: A psychiatric study of 247 liver transplantation candidates. Psychosomatics 30:147–153, 1989

Trzepacz PT, Levenson JL, Tringali RA: Psychopharmacology and neuropsychiatric syndrome in organ transplantation. Gen Hosp Psychiatry 13:233–245, 1991

Twillman RK, Manetto C, Wellisch DK, et al: The Transplant Evaluation Rating Scale: a revision of the psychosocial levels system for evaluating organ transplant candidates. Psychosomatics 34:144–153, 1993

Vaillant GE, Clark W, Cyrus C, et al: Prospective study of alcoholism treatment: eight-year follow-up. Am J Med 75:455–463, 1983

Valldeoriola F, Graus F, Rimola A, et al: Cyclosporine-associated mutism in liver transplant patients. Neurology 46:252–254, 1996

Vella J, Sayegh M: Interactions between cyclosporine and newer antidepressant medications. Am J Kidney Dis 31:320–323, 1998

Wang WL, Yang ZF, Lo CM, et al: Intracerebral hemorrhage after liver transplantation. Liver Transpl 6:345–348, 2000

Wijdicks EFM, Blue PR, Steers JL, et al: Central pontine myelinolysis with stupor alone after orthotopic liver transplantation. Liver Transpl Surg 2:14–16, 1996

Wilt JL, Minnema AM, Johnson RF, et al: Torsades de pointes associated with the use of intravenous haloperidol. Ann Intern Med 119:391–394, 1993

Wise MG, Trzepacz PT: Delirium (confusional states), in The American Psychiatric Press Textbook of Consultation-Liaison Psychiatry. Edited by Rundell JR, Wise MG. Washington, DC, American Psychiatric Press, 1996, pp 258–274

Woodman CL, Geist LJ, Vance S, et al: Psychiatric disorders and survival after lung transplantation. Psychosomatics 40:293–297, 1999

Yates WR, Booth BM, Reed DA, et al: Descriptive and predictive ability of a high-risk alcoholism relapse model. J Stud Alcohol 54:645–651, 1993

Yates WR, LaBrecque DR, Pfab D: Personality disorder as a contraindication for liver transplantation in alcoholic cirrhosis. Psychosomatics 39:501–511, 1998

Chapter 4

Psychiatric Disorders and the Menstrual Cycle

Laura J. Miller, M.D.

Introduction: The Nature of Menstruation

The monthly hormonal flux and shedding of blood that constitutes the human menstrual cycle is a relatively recent evolutionary development (Strassmann 1996). As a system, it seems by design to be responsive to social and environmental context. For example, the endocrinological transformations leading to menarche are triggered by leptin, a hormone secreted by fat cells. This ensures that only girls who are sufficiently well nourished will become fertile (Hrdy 1999). Menarche also happens earlier, independent of weight, in girls whose families have high levels of conflict and whose fathers are absent (Moffitt et al. 1992). Once menstruation has begun, stress and/or malnutrition can suppress it. It is posited that the system evolved to shut down under adverse conditions for bearing young and to appear under optimal or necessary conditions. Because of this, the neuroendocrine systems influencing hunger, stress responses, affiliative feelings, and reproduction are closely intertwined and mutually regulatory.

Given the interconnections between reproductive hormones and stress hormones, it is not surprising that menstruation can become linked to changes in mood and behavior. Although mood changes across the cycle are not universal (Laessle et al. 1990), some women note regularly cycling differences in mood, and a subset of these women experience clinically significant dysphoria premenstrually. In this chapter, I summarize data about the etiology and treatment of these premenstrual mood disorders.

Premenstrual Psychiatric Disorders

Premenstrual mood changes were defined as a syndrome in 1931, when both Horney and Frank published accounts of "premenstrual tension" (Richardson 1995). In 1953, Greene and Dalton broadened this concept and proposed the term *premenstrual syndrome* (PMS) for psychiatric and physical symptoms that regularly occur premenstrually. This term continues to be widely used. However, there was a lack of consensus about the severity of symptoms, degree of symptom change from one cycle phase to another, type of symptoms, and level of functional impairment implied by this designation (Spitzer et al. 1989). To distinguish a clinically meaningful syndrome from milder premenstrual changes, DSM-III-R (American Psychiatric Association 1987) included a working definition of "late luteal phase dysphoric disorder." This was subsequently changed to "premenstrual dysphoric disorder" (PMDD) in DSM-IV (American Psychiatric Association 1994). Symptoms of PMDD, along with illustrative descriptions from a study of the narrative portion of the Premenstrual Assessment Form (Cumming et al. 1994), can include

- Depressed mood and hopelessness: "I feel a failure…nothing I can do will change that."
- Anxiety or tension: "3–5 days are filled with…extreme anxiety."
- Affective lability: "Life is like a roller coaster ride."
- Irritability: "I tend to flare up at my children, 'bark' at my husband more.…"
- Anhedonia: "I can't see any reason to go to work, dress up for anything.…"
- Poor concentration: "Body present, mind is very cloudy, almost like dream world."
- Fatigue or lack of energy: "sluggish…tired, low energy…"
- Change in appetite: "urge to eat anything and everything—a real binge."
- Sleep disturbance: "Want to go to sleep forever (not a suicidal thought, just a measure of fatigue)."
- Feeling overwhelmed: "overly upset over little problems while normally little problems do not bother me."
- Physical symptoms: "pelvic heaviness and feeling bloated."

By definition, women with PMDD have five or more of the above symptoms during the last week of the luteal phase of the menstrual cycle. Symptoms begin to remit within a few days after the onset of the follicular phase and are gone by a week after menses onset. Symptoms occur during most or all menstrual cycles and interfere with social and/or occupational functioning.

Defined in this way, PMDD is present in about 5% of the samples of non-treatment-seeking women (Rivera-Tovar and Frank 1990) and in about 14%–45% of women seeking treatment in PMS clinics (Hurt et al. 1992). Symptoms usually remain similar from cycle to cycle (Bloch et al. 1997) and persist over many years (Roca et al. 1999). Having premenstrual mood changes increases the likelihood of experiencing peripartum depression (Sugawara et al. 1997) and perimenopausal dysphoria (Morse et al. 1998).

Some women have psychiatric symptoms throughout their menstrual cycles, but their symptoms intensify premenstrually. This pattern of premenstrual exacerbation has been noted for several psychiatric disorders, including major depression (Yonkers 1997b), dysthymic disorder (Endicott 1993), bipolar disorder (Brockington et al. 1988), panic disorder (Yonkers 1997a), generalized anxiety disorder (McLeod et al. 1993), schizoaffective disorder (Sothern et al. 1993), and schizophrenia (Levitte 1997).

At times, premenstrual symptoms become apparent after treatment alleviates symptoms in the rest of the menstrual cycle. Sometimes premenstrual symptom persistence after pharmacotherapy does not reflect a true exacerbation but is due to differences in drug availability across the menstrual cycle. Hormonal influences on pharmacokinetics are of sufficient magnitude in some women that serum levels of some mood-stabilizing and antidepressant medications differ across the menstrual cycle at constant oral doses (Jensvold et al. 1992). In most such cases, serum levels are lower in the luteal phase than in the follicular phase.

Because many relevant research studies, even those with carefully defined entry criteria, have not used the formal DSM-IV definition of PMDD, I use the more general term *PMS* when summarizing findings.

Premenstrual Syndrome: Contributory Factors

Genetic

Available data support the idea that there is a genetic susceptibility to PMS. Monozygotic twins' scores on PMS questionnaires correlate significantly more with each other than do the scores for dizygotic twins (Condon 1993; Kendler et al. 1998). In Kendler and colleagues' twin study, the model that best fit the data was that both genetic and environmental factors played a major role in vulnerability to PMS. Heritability of PMS was estimated to be about 56%. Other investigators pointed out, however, that a general tendency to report complaints might be heritable and might account for the increased reporting of PMS symptoms in monozygotic compared with dizygotic twins (Van den Akker et al. 1995).

Neuroendocrine

Most studies have found that circulating levels of gonadotropins and gonadal hormones are not significantly different in women with PMS as compared with asymptomatic women (Rubinow and Schmidt 1995). A few studies have found abnormalities in the stress-responsive hypothalamic-pituitary-adrenal (HPA) axis in women with PMS, but findings have been contradictory, and study participant pools have been small (Bloch et al. 1998; Odber et al. 1998; Rabin et al. 1990; Rosenstein et al. 1996).

A more consistent picture is beginning to emerge from studies of key neurotransmitters that are modulated by reproductive hormones. Estrogen and progesterone influence serotonin synthesis and metabolism (Halbreich and Tworek 1993). In women without PMS or PMDD, plasma serotonin levels rise during the luteal phase and decline during the follicular phase of the menstrual cycle (Blum et al. 1992; Hindberg and Naesh 1992). In women with PMDD, both state and trait serotonergic abnormalities have been found, including decreased luteal phase serotonin levels and blunted responses to serotonergic challenge tests (Kouri and Halbreich 1997).

A central role in the etiology of PMS has been posited for the inhibitory, anxiolytic neurotransmitter γ-aminobutyric acid (GABA). During the symptomatic late luteal phase of the menstrual cycle, women with PMS have been found to have significantly lower plasma GABA levels (Halbreich et al. 1996) and functional sensitivity to GABA agonists (Sundstrom et al. 1997) than do control subjects. During the asymptomatic follicular phase, GABA levels and functional sensitivity to GABA agonists are comparable in women with PMS and healthy control subjects.

GABA's role in PMS may be mediated by the neuroactive progesterone metabolites pregnanolone and allopregnanolone. These compounds are synthesized in the ovaries and in the brain and can rapidly alter central nervous system excitability (Morrow et al. 1995). They act primarily as GABA-A agonists but also may act directly on the HPA axis. During the follicular phase, the levels of these neuroactive steroids and the functional sensitivity to them are comparable in women with and without PMS. However, during the symptomatic luteal phase, women with PMS have been found to have significantly lower levels of allopregnanolone (Rapkin et al. 1997). Also during the luteal phase, women with PMS have been found to be significantly less sensitive to pregnanolone injections than are women without PMS (Sundstrom et al. 1998). During menstrual cycles in which pregnanolone and allopregnanolone levels are lowest, women with PMS report significantly more depression and fatigue (Wang et al. 1996).

Psychological

To date, no data clearly show preexisting personality characteristics that constitute risk factors for developing PMS. In fact, measures of personality traits that have been thought to be stable over time, such as the Minnesota Multiphasic Personality Inventory and Locus of Control, have been shown to vary across the menstrual cycle in women with PMS (O'Boyle et al. 1988; Palmer et al. 1991).

Personality disorders, as defined in DSM-IV-TR (American Psychiatric Association 2000), generally have not been found with greater frequency in women with PMS than in women without PMS. Avoidant personality disorder may be an exception. However, in a study that compared women by age groups, an association between PMS and avoidant personality disorder was found only for women older than 30 years (De Ronchi et al. 2000). This suggests that avoidant traits did not precede and predispose to PMS but that PMS may lead to avoidant behavior over time.

Some investigators have questioned whether negative expectations about premenstrual experience influence women to report premenstrual symptoms. However, when awareness of study focus was systematically manipulated, no evidence indicated that women who knew the study was about PMS reported more premenstrual dysphoria than did women who did not know this (Gallant et al. 1991).

Sociocultural

Sociocultural context has been posited to affect PMS in two major ways. One is that cultural practices strongly influence a woman's lifetime menstrual pattern. In societies in which artificial contraception is not used and prolonged breast-feeding is practiced, women have many fewer menstrual cycles over the course of their reproductive lives (Strassman 1996). A second posited influence is that negative cultural attitudes about menstruation could influence women's expectations of premenstrual dysphoria. In North America and Great Britain, where most of the PMS studies have taken place, media portrayal of the menstrual cycle is associated with shame and stigma (Coutts and Berg 1993), and media accounts of PMS are often exaggerated and wildly inaccurate (Chrisler and Levy 1990). Nevertheless, premenstrual dysphoria has been reported in a wide variety of cultures, including cultures in which less media attention is given to PMS (Sveinsdottir 1998). A study comparing women of different religious beliefs, including religions with and without specific menstrual prohibitions, found that religion had little effect on attitudes toward menstruation or on the reporting of symptoms related to the menstrual cycle (Rothbaum and Jackson 1990).

Premenstrual Syndrome: Treatment

Pharmacotherapy

Antidepressants

Of all the interventions posited to alleviate premenstrual dysphoria, antidepressants with serotonergic activity have the most robust evidence of efficacy. Numerous well-designed trials have confirmed the superiority of serotonergic antidepressants (e.g., selective serotonin reuptake inhibitors [SSRIs] and clomipramine) over placebo in alleviating the symptoms of PMDD (Dimmock et al. 2000). SSRI antidepressants are significantly more effective than antidepressants with less or no serotonergic activity (e.g., maprotiline, bupropion, or desipramine) (Eriksson et al. 1995; Freeman et al. 1999b; Pearlstein et al. 1997); the latter are not significantly different from placebo in their effects on PMDD. An open-label study of nefazodone, an agent that is less selectively serotonergic but produces some serotonin type 2 receptor antagonism and serotonin reuptake inhibition, also significantly reduced premenstrual dysphoria (Freeman et al. 1994). For women with PMDD who experience sexual dysfunction and insomnia from SSRIs, nefazodone may prove to be a viable alternative treatment.

Relatively low antidepressant doses suffice for most women with PMDD. For fluoxetine, doses as low as 10 mg/day have shown efficacy (Diegoli et al. 1998), whereas 60 mg appeared to confer no advantage over 20 mg/day (Steiner et al. 1995). Effective ranges for other antidepressants have been as follows: sertraline, 50–150 mg/day (Freeman et al. 1999b; Yonkers et al. 1997); paroxetine, 10–30 mg/day (Eriksson et al. 1995); and clomipramine, 25–75 mg/day (Sundblad et al. 1992).

Luteal phase dosing is the practice of using medication for PMS only during the symptomatic luteal phase of the menstrual cycle. A typical luteal phase dosing regimen begins at about the time of ovulation, 14 days before the anticipated onset of menses in a 28-day cycle. Medication is discontinued at or shortly after menses onset and resumes on day 14 of the subsequent cycle. Luteal phase dosing has been shown to be significantly more effective than placebo (Halbreich and Smoller 1997; Jermain et al.

1999; Steiner et al. 1997; Sundblad et al. 1993; Young et al. 1998). In a study directly comparing luteal phase dosing with continuous dosing of sertraline, luteal phase dosing was significantly more effective (Freeman et al. 1999a). It is possible that this is because this dosing pattern mimics more closely the natural peaks and valleys of serotonin and GABA that occur during the normal menstrual cycle. Although it has not yet been systematically studied, a case report suggested that fluoxetine, because of its long half-life, may be effective when used only once per cycle on the first day of symptom onset (Daamen and Brown 1992).

The efficacy of these dosing regimens may seem to contradict studies that show that antidepressants take several weeks to achieve optimal effects. However, SSRI antidepressants have been shown to rapidly increase functional sensitivity to GABA agonists in women with PMS (Sundstrom and Backstrom 1998); this may explain their prompt effectiveness.

Although dosing only during the symptomatic phase of the cycle could reduce side effects, it could increase side effects as well because of repeated acclimation and withdrawal. This has been observed for clomipramine (Sundblad et al. 1993) but not for SSRIs to date (Freeman et al. 1999a). The on-off side effects of clomipramine can be minimized by the use of a luteal phase boosting regimen. For example, a small dose (5–10 mg/day) can alternate with a higher dose (25–75 mg/day) during the luteal phase (Sundblad et al. 1993).

Available data suggest that long-term use of antidepressants for PMDD is indicated and effective (Menkes et al. 1992, 1993). For women whose premenstrual dysphoria is markedly intensified during the fall and winter months, some clinicians vary antidepressant doses across the seasons of the year. There are no systematic studies to date of this form of chronotherapy.

Anxiolytics

Because anxiety is a prominent premenstrual symptom for many women, investigators have studied the efficacy of anxiolytic agents for treating PMS. Among the benzodiazepines, the best studied for this indication is alprazolam. Findings have been equivocal, with some studies reporting greater effectiveness than placebo (Harrison et al. 1990) and some finding no difference from placebo (Schmidt et al. 1993). Doses have ranged from 0.25 to 5.0 mg/day, with many women experiencing sedation at higher doses. This may account for some of the variance in study findings; the dropout rate increases at higher doses, and efficacy may be less at lower doses. Alprazolam has been used in a luteal phase dosing pattern but only if tapered by no more than 25% per day beginning at menses onset (Harrison et al. 1990). Abrupt discontinuation can cause anxiety, palpitations, tremors, and seizures. Because of its rapid onset of action, alprazolam can be used on an as-needed basis for occasional symptomatic days or while women are charting their symptoms for diagnostic purposes before treatment.

Buspirone, a nonbenzodiazepine anxiolytic agent, has been less well studied but also has been shown to reduce symptoms of PMS (Rickels et al. 1989). The mechanism of action of buspirone is unknown, but its serotonin type 1A receptor agonist activity has been posited to account for its efficacy for PMS. Buspirone has been used for this purpose in a dose range of 15–60 mg/day in either continuous or luteal phase dosing patterns.

Spironolactone

Spironolactone is a diuretic that inhibits aldosterone and certain effects of angiotensin. It also has antiandrogenic properties and decreases serum levels of progesterone while increasing estradiol. Some, but not all, double-blind studies have found it to be significantly more effective than placebo in decreasing PMS symptoms (Burnet et al. 1991; Hellberg et al. 1991; Wang et al. 1995). Because other diuretics do not alleviate PMS, it is posited that spironolactone's hormonal actions account for its efficacy. It is usually given in a dose of 100 mg/day during the luteal phase.

Diet

Although some investigators have suggested various nutritional deficiencies or excesses as causes of PMS, no convincing evidence of this exists (Chuong and Dawson 1992). Nevertheless, specific dietary modifications can help alleviate premenstrual symptoms.

The nutritional interventions with the most evidence of efficacy are calcium supplementation, complex carbohydrates, and reduction of alcohol consumption.

Calcium

Diets low in calcium can worsen mood and concentration throughout the menstrual cycle, even in healthy women without PMS (Penland and Johnson 1993). The activity of calcium-regulating hormones fluctuates across the menstrual cycle, and these fluctuations may be exaggerated in women with PMS (Thys-Jacobs and Alvir 1995). These observations have led some investigators to posit that calcium supplementation could alleviate PMS. A randomized, double-blind study found that women with PMS who were treated with calcium supplementation (1,200 mg/day) had significantly fewer luteal phase symptoms than did those who received placebo (Thys-Jacobs et al. 1998). Calcium supplementation reduced negative affect, food cravings, pain, and water retention. No significant difference between calcium and placebo in their effects on mood was seen during other menstrual cycle phases.

As a therapeutic agent, calcium has the advantages of being relatively inexpensive, having relatively few side effects, and conferring protection against osteoporosis. Most menstruating women in the United States have a mean daily calcium intake in the 600–800 mg range (Bendich 2000), which is considerably lower than the 1,200 mg shown to alleviate PMS. A potential long-term adverse effect of calcium supplementation is the buildup of calcium oxalate renal stones, although this does not usually occur unless doses exceed 2,500 mg/day. Taking calcium supplements with meals can reduce this risk because this will bind some dietary oxalate, reducing its absorption and renal excretion.

Carbohydrates

Craving of carbohydrate-rich foods is a common symptom premenstrually, especially in the presence of depressed mood (Dye et al. 1995). Under controlled conditions, women with PMS were shown to increase their daily food intake by as much as 500 calories during the late luteal phase (Wurtman 1990). Most of the increased intake was in the form of carbohydrates. Women without PMS did not have changes in their total calorie or nutrient intake across the menstrual cycle.

Some evidence suggests that carbohydrate craving represents a physiological mechanism to increase serotonin in the brain. Certain types of carbohydrates facilitate the uptake of tryptophan, the amino acid precursor of serotonin, into the brain. By contrast, protein-rich foods supply other amino acids that compete with tryptophan for binding sites and decrease its uptake (Wurtman 1990). A double-blind crossover trial found that a tryptophan-enhancing carbohydrate beverage improved mood significantly more than did placebo beverages (a protein drink and a non-tryptophan-enhancing carbohydrate drink) in women with PMS (Sayegh et al. 1995). By choosing lower-fat carbohydrate-rich foods, and compensating for premenstrual caloric increases with aerobic exercise, women can take advantage of the mood-enhancing properties of carbohydrates without compromising their general health status.

Alcoholic Beverage Reduction

Some evidence indicates that women with PMS drink significantly more alcoholic beverages than do women without PMS (Caan et al. 1993). Among women with PMS, the desire for alcohol was found to be significantly higher premenstrually than during other cycle phases (Evans et al. 1999). Heavy alcohol drinking is associated with a significantly higher risk of physical menstrual abnormalities, such as heavy menstrual bleeding (Kritz-Silverstein et al. 1999). Although no direct evidence to date shows that reducing alcohol intake specifically improves PMS symptoms, ample evidence suggests that heavy drinking increases dysphoric mood states in general. Therefore, countering the extra alcohol cravings conferred by PMS is likely to improve dysphoria. If antidepressant medications are prescribed, simultaneously eliminating alcoholic beverages may become easier to do and may reduce medication side effects.

Exercise

Exercise alleviates premenstrual physical and emotional symptoms (Aganoff and Boyle 1994; Steege and Blumenthal 1993). Aerobic exercise appears to be more effective than strength training for decreasing premenstrual depression. Because exercise improves adaptation to stress regardless of menstrual cycle phase (Choi and Salmon 1995), the therapeutic effects of exercise may not be specific for PMS. However, because exercise acutely raises serum progesterone levels, it is possible (although not proven) that exercise favorably alters cyclic hormonal patterns (Steege and Blumenthal 1993).

Psychotherapy

Cognitive-behavioral therapy, interpersonal therapy, and psychoeducational therapy have been found to be effective in alleviating premenstrual dysphoric symptoms. Some women with PMS have anticipatory anxiety before their symptoms occur, which can heighten sensitivity to premenstrual changes. Some experience a sense of helplessness when faced with cyclic change that feels out of their control. Cognitive therapy approaches focus on diminishing anticipatory anxiety and combating helpless feelings. Behavioral approaches include limiting controllable stressors at vulnerable times (e.g., not planning deadlines or difficult meetings premenstrually) (Reading 1992). A structured psychoeducational approach, including relaxation training, assertiveness training, and parenting training, also has been effective (Christensen and Oei 1995).

Phototherapy

Bright-light therapy, as compared with a placebo condition of dim red-light exposure, has been shown to significantly improve symptoms of PMS (Lam et al. 1999). The reason for its efficacy is unknown. Disturbances in circadian patterns have been noted in women with PMS (Parry et al. 1994); phototherapy may normalize these disturbances. A substantial portion of women with PMS note seasonal worsening of their premenstrual symptoms (Maskall et al. 1997). Some women have premenstrual symptoms only during the fall and winter months (Parry et al. 1987). Phototherapy may be particularly effective for women with seasonal exacerbations of PMS, although it may have some efficacy even in the absence of seasonal patterns.

When phototherapy is prescribed, patients can be instructed to use a light box emitting 10,000 lux cool-white fluorescent light and filtering out ultraviolet light. Patients are asked to sit in front of the light box, about 3 feet from its face, for 30 minutes daily and to glance toward the box every few seconds.

Hormonal Interventions

Gonadotropin-Releasing Hormone Analogues

During normal menstrual cycles, gonadotropin-releasing hormone (GnRH) from the pituitary gland orchestrates many of the hormonal events. Giving exogenous GnRH analogues initially causes an increase in gonadotropins, but after 1–2 weeks, continuous exposure suppresses ovulation, inducing reversible "chemical menopause." In most, but not all, women with PMS, this alleviates symptoms (Schmidt et al. 1998). Long-term use can accelerate the medical risks associated with menopause, such as osteoporosis. Adding back estrogen (along with progesterone to reduce the risk of endometrial cancer) can reduce these risks. Unfortunately, replacing estrogen and/or progesterone usually brings back some of the PMS symptoms (Muse 1992; Schmidt et al. 1998). One promising regimen has used low-dose add-back therapy without producing symptom recurrence (Mezrow et al. 1994). Leuprolide acetate (a GnRH analogue) was given every 4 weeks as a 7.5-mg intramuscular injection. When the women began to experience estrogen-deficiency symptoms (e.g., hot flashes, vaginal dryness), conjugated equine estrogen was given at a dose of 0.625 mg 6 days per week. Medroxyprogesterone acetate was given at a dose of 10 mg/day for 10 days every four menstrual cycles. Improvement in PMS symptoms continued over the study duration of 12 months. This treatment may be effective for some women, but it is costly, complicated, and relatively invasive. Its long-term safety has yet to be studied, especially with regard to effects on bone density and risk of endometrial cancer. It is worth considering for women with severe PMS whose symptoms are not responsive to other treatments.

Danazol

Danazol is a synthetic derivative of $17\text{-}\alpha\text{-ethinyltestosterone}$. Its pharmacological actions include suppressing mid-cycle follicle-stimulating hormone and luteinizing hormone surges, inhibiting the synthesis of gonadal steroids, and binding to gonadal steroid receptors. Low-dose danazol (e.g., 100 mg twice a day) has been found to be significantly superior to placebo in alleviating symptoms of PMS (Deeny et al. 1991). At that dose, danazol suppresses ovulation in some, but not all, women. It can be effective with luteal phase dosing as well, in which case it does not suppress ovulation (Sarno et al. 1987).

Danazol's side effects include weight gain, irregular menses, acne, and depression. Used at a higher dose (200 mg twice a day), danazol was not significantly different from placebo in alleviating depressed mood in women with PMS (Hahn et al. 1995). Depression as a side effect may be more likely at higher doses, counteracting whatever therapeutic benefit might have been conferred at lower doses. Danazol may be useful for women with PMS who need it for other indications simultaneously (e.g., endometriosis or mastalgia), but side effects limit its usefulness for many women.

Hysterectomy

Hysterectomy with bilateral oophorectomy eliminates ovulatory menstrual cycling and often eliminates PMS. For some women, postoperative hormone replacement therapy causes symptom recurrence (Henshaw et al. 1996). Because of the risks of the surgery, combined with the risks of premature menopause, this is a treatment of last resort, usually used only when another indication for hysterectomy is present. Hysterectomy that leaves one or both ovaries intact seems to alleviate PMS for some, but not all, women (Braiden and Metcalf 1995). This appears to be the case even in women who feel that they can tell when they are ovulating posthysterectomy.

Treatments That Are Probably Ineffective

Evening Primrose Oil

One hypothesis about the cause of PMS is that affected women have low levels of omega-6 essential fatty acids. Because these essential fatty acids are prostaglandin precursors, this relative deficiency is posited to cause abnormalities in prostaglandin synthesis that, in turn, cause premenstrual symptoms. Based on this idea, evening primrose oil has become a popular herbal treatment for PMS. Evening primrose oil contains a high concentration of γ-linolenic acid. Although it has few side effects, evening primrose oil is probably not an effective treatment for PMS. Although some trials found that evening primrose oil significantly reduced PMS symptoms as compared with placebo, these trials had significant methodological flaws. Two relatively small but well-controlled studies did not find any significant difference between evening primrose oil and placebo effects on PMS (Budeiri et al. 1996).

Pyridoxine (Vitamin B$_6$)

High-dose pyridoxine (usually 50–500 mg/day, as compared with the recommended daily allowance of 2 mg/day) has been recommended as a treatment for PMS. The primary rationale is that its active form, pyridoxal 5'phosphate, is a cofactor in the metabolic pathways of several neurotransmitters, including serotonin. The aggregate findings of several randomized, double-blind, placebo-controlled trials of pyridoxine did not support its efficacy as a treatment for PMS (Kleijnen et al. 1990).

Oral Contraceptive Pills

Because oral contraceptive pills suppress ovulation and alter hormonal cyclicity, it has been posited that they can treat PMS. However, women with PMS have reported highly varied effects from oral contraceptive pills. In a survey of women with PMS who had used oral contraception since becoming symptomatic, 31% felt that oral contraceptive pills had alleviated PMS symptoms, 20% reported that oral contraceptive pills had worsened PMS symptoms, 32% saw no difference with oral contraceptive pills, and 17% did not know (Corney and Stanton 1991). Comparisons of women with PMS who use combined oral contraceptive pills, triphasic oral contraceptive pills, and no oral contraceptive pills showed no significant differences in the severity of premenstrual mood symptoms among these three groups (Bancroft and Rennie 1993).

Progesterone

Progesterone has been the most widely used hormonal intervention for PMS. Because its oral absorption is poor, it usually has been given by vaginal suppository. Despite its popularity, several double-blind studies have not found that progesterone is any better than placebo in alleviating symptoms of PMS (Muse 1992).

Conclusion

Clinically significant premenstrual mood changes affect about 5% of menstruating women, and many women with Axis I psychiatric disorders experience premenstrual symptom exacerbation. Vulnerability to premenstrual dysphoria appears to be partly heritable and to be based in part on interactions between reproductive hormones and the neurotransmitters serotonin and GABA. -PMDD or premenstrual exacerbation can be diagnosed by prospectively charting symptoms across the menstrual cycle and by interviewing the patient during different phases of the cycle. A comprehensive treatment approach for most women includes serotonergic antidepressants (using luteal phase dosing when indicated), targeted psychotherapy, calcium supplementation, and aerobic exercise. For selected patients, treatment with anxiolytic medication, spironolactone, GnRH analogues, danazol, or phototherapy also may be effective.

References

Aganoff JA, Boyle GJ: Aerobic exercise, mood states and menstrual cycle symptoms. J Psychosom Res 38:183–192, 1994

American Psychiatric Association: Diagnostic and Statistical Manual of Mental Disorders, 3rd Edition, Revised. Washington, DC, American Psychiatric Association, 1987

American Psychiatric Association: Diagnostic and Statistical Manual of Mental Disorders, 4th Edition. Washington, DC, American Psychiatric Association, 1994

American Psychiatric Association: Diagnostic and Statistical Manual of Mental Disorders, 4th Edition, Text Revision. Washington, DC, American Psychiatric Association, 2000

Bancroft J, Rennie D: The impact of oral contraceptives on the experience of perimenstrual mood, clumsiness, food craving and other symptoms. J Psychosom Res 37:195–202, 1993

Bendich A: The potential for dietary supplements to reduce premenstrual syndrome (PMS) symptoms. J Am Coll Nutr 19:3–12, 2000

Bloch M, Schmidt PJ, Rubinow DR: Premenstrual syndrome: evidence for symptom stability across cycles. Am J Psychiatry 154:1741–1746, 1997

Bloch M, Schmidt PJ, Su TP, et al: Pituitary-adrenal hormones and testosterone across the menstrual cycle in women with premenstrual syndrome and controls. Biol Psychiatry 43:897–903, 1998

Blum I, Nessiel L, David A, et al: Plasma neurotransmitter profile during different phases of the ovulatory cycle. J Clin Endocrinol Metab 75:924–929, 1992

Braiden V, Metcalf G: Premenstrual tension among hysterectomized women. J Psychosom Obstet Gynaecol 16:145–151, 1995

Brockington IF, Kelly A, Hall P, et al: Premenstrual relapse of puerperal psychosis. J Affect Disord 14:287–292, 1988

Budeiri D, Po ALW, Dornan JC: Is evening primrose oil of value in the treatment of premenstrual syndrome? Control Clin Trials 17:60–68, 1996

Burnet RB, Radden HS, Esterbrook EG, et al: Premenstrual syndrome and spironolactone. Aust N Z J Obstet Gynaecol 31:366–368, 1991

Caan B, Duncan D, Hiatt R, et al: Association between alcoholic and caffeinated beverages and premenstrual syndrome. J Reprod Med 38:630–636, 1993

Choi PYL, Salmon P: Stress responsivity in exercisers and non-exercisers during different phases of the menstrual cycle. Soc Sci Med 41:769–777, 1995

Chrisler JC, Levy KB: The media construct a menstrual monster: a content analysis of PMS articles in the popular press. Women Health 16:89–104, 1990

Christensen AP, Oei TPS: The efficacy of cognitive behavior therapy in treating premenstrual dysphoric changes. J Affect Disord 33:57–63, 1995

Chuong CJ, Dawson EB: Critical evaluation of nutritional factors in the pathophysiology and treatment of premenstrual syndrome. Clin Obstet Gynecol 35:679–692, 1992

Condon JT: The premenstrual syndrome: a twin study. Br J Psychiatry 162:481–486, 1993

Corney RH, Stanton R: A survey of 658 women who report symptoms of premenstrual syndrome. J Psychosom Res 35:471–482, 1991

Coutts LB, Berg DH: The portrayal of the menstruating woman in menstrual product advertisements. Health Care Women Int 14:179–191, 1993

Cumming CE, Urion C, Cumming DC, et al: "So mean and cranky, I could bite my mother": an ethnosemantic analysis of women's descriptions of premenstrual change. Women Health 21:21–41, 1994

Daamen MJ, Brown WA: Single-dose fluoxetine in management of premenstrual syndrome (letter). J Clin Psychiatry 53:210–211, 1992

De Ronchi D, Muro A, Marziani A, et al: Personality disorders and depressive symptoms in late luteal phase dysphoric disorder. Psychother Psychosom 69:27–34, 2000

Deeny M, Hawthorn R, Hart DM: Low dose danazol in the treatment of the premenstrual syndrome. Postgrad Med J 67:450–454, 1991

Diegoli MSC, da Fonseca AM, Diegoli CA, et al: A double-blind trial of four medications to treat severe premenstrual syndrome. Int J Gynaecol Obstet 62:63–67, 1998

Dimmock PW, Wyatt KM, Jones PW, et al: Efficacy of selective serotonin-reuptake inhibitors in premenstrual syndrome: a systematic review. Lancet 356:1131–1136, 2000

Dye L, Warner P, Bancroft J: Food craving during the menstrual cycle and its relationship to stress, happiness of relationship and depression; a preliminary enquiry. J Affect Disord 34:157–164, 1995

Endicott J: The menstrual cycle and mood disorders. J Affect Disord 29:193–200, 1993

Eriksson E, Hedberg MA, Andersch B, et al: The serotonin reuptake inhibitor paroxetine is superior to the noradrenaline reuptake inhibitor maprotiline in the treatment of premenstrual syndrome. Neuropsychopharmacology 12:167–176, 1995

Evans SM, Foltin RW, Fischman MW: Food "cravings" and the acute effects of alprazolam on food intake in women with premenstrual dysphoric disorder. Appetite 32:331–349, 1999

Freeman EW, Rickels K, Sondheimer SJ, et al: Nefazodone in the treatment of premenstrual syndrome: a preliminary study. J Clin Psychopharmacol 14:180–186, 1994

Freeman EW, Rickels K, Arredondo F, et al: Full- or half-cycle treatment of severe premenstrual syndrome with a serotonergic antidepressant. J Clin Psychopharmacol 19:3–8, 1999a

Freeman EW, Rickels K, Sondheimer SJ, et al: Differential response to antidepressants in women with premenstrual syndrome/premenstrual dysphoric disorder: a randomized controlled trial. Arch Gen Psychiatry 56:932–939, 1999b

Gallant SJ, Hamilton JA, Popiel DA, et al: Daily moods and symptoms: effects of awareness of study focus, gender, menstrual-cycle phase, and day of the week. Health Psychol 10:180–189, 1991

Greene R, Dalton K: The premenstrual syndrome. BMJ 1:1007–1014, 1953

Hahn PM, Van Vugt DA, Reid RL: A randomized, placebo-controlled, crossover trial of danazol for the treatment of premenstrual syndrome. Psychoneuroendocrinology 20:193–209, 1995

Halbreich U, Smoller JW: Intermittent luteal phase sertraline treatment of dysphoric premenstrual syndrome. J Clin Psychiatry 58:399–402, 1997

Halbreich U, Tworek H: Altered serotonergic activity in women with dysphoric premenstrual syndromes. Int J Psychiatry Med 23:1–27, 1993

Halbreich U, Petty F, Yonkers K, et al: Low plasma gamma-aminobutyric acid levels during the late luteal phase of women with premenstrual dysphoric disorder. Am J Psychiatry 153:718–720, 1996

Harrison WM, Endicott J, Nee J: Treatment of premenstrual dysphoria with alprazolam: a controlled study. Arch Gen Psychiatry 47:270–275, 1990

Hellberg D, Claesson B, Nilsson S: Premenstrual tension: a placebo-controlled efficacy study with spironolactone and medroxyprogesterone acetate. Int J Gynaecol Obstet 34:243–248, 1991

Henshaw C, Foreman D, Belcher J, et al: Can one induce premenstrual symptomatology in women with prior hysterectomy and bilateral oophorectomy? J Psychosom Obstet Gynaecol 17:21–28, 1996

Hindberg I, Naesh O: Serotonin concentrations in plasma and variations during the menstrual cycle. Clin Chem 38:2087–2089, 1992

Hrdy SB: Mother Nature: A History of Mothers, Infants, and Natural Selection. New York, Pantheon, 1999, p 125

Hurt SW, Schnurr PP, Severino SK, et al: Late luteal phase dysphoric disorder in 670 women evaluated for premenstrual complaints. Am J Psychiatry 149:525–530, 1992

Jensvold MF, Reed K, Jarrett DB, et al: Menstrual cycle-related depressive symptoms treated with variable antidepressant dosage. J Womens Health 1:109–115, 1992

Jermain DM, Preece CK, Sykes RL, et al: Luteal phase sertraline treatment for premenstrual dysphoric disorder: results of a double-blind, placebo-controlled, crossover study. Arch Fam Med 8:328–332, 1999

Kendler KS, Karkowski LM, Corey LA, et al: Longitudinal population-based twin study of retrospectively reported premenstrual symptoms and lifetime major depression. Am J Psychiatry 155:1234–1240, 1998

Kleijnen J, Riet GT, Knipschild P: Vitamin B6 in the treatment of the premenstrual syndrome—a review. Br J Obstet Gynaecol 97:847–852, 1990

Kouri EM, Halbreich U: State and trait serotonergic abnormalities in women with dysphoric premenstrual syndromes. Psychopharmacol Bull 33:767–770, 1997

Kritz-Silverstein D, Wingard DL, Garland FC: The association of behavior and lifestyle factors with menstrual symptoms. Journal of Women's Health and Gender-Based Medicine 8:1185–1193, 1999

Laessle RG, Tuschl RJ, Schweiger U, et al: Mood changes and physical complaints during the normal menstrual cycle in healthy young women. Psychoneuroendocrinology 15:131–138, 1990

Lam RW, Carter D, Misri S, et al: A controlled study of light therapy in women with late luteal phase dysphoric disorder. Psychiatry Res 86:185–192, 1999

Levitte SS: Treatment of premenstrual exacerbation of schizophrenia. Psychosomatics 38:582–584, 1997

Maskall DD, Lam RW, Misri S, et al: Seasonality of symptoms in women with late luteal phase dysphoric disorder. Am J Psychiatry 154:1436–1441, 1997

McLeod DR, Hoehn-Saric R, Fostre GV, et al: The influence of premenstrual syndrome on ratings of anxiety in women with generalized anxiety disorder. Acta Psychiatr Scand 88:248–251, 1993

Menkes DB, Taghavi E, Mason PA, et al: Fluoxetine treatment of severe premenstrual syndrome. BMJ 305:346–347, 1992

Menkes DB, Taghavi E, Mason PA, et al: Fluoxetine's spectrum of action in premenstrual syndrome. Int Clin Psychopharmacol 8:95–102, 1993

Mezrow G, Shoupe D, Spicer D, et al: Depot leuprolide acetate with estrogen and progestin add-back for long-term treatment of premenstrual syndrome. Fertil Steril 62:932–937, 1994

Moffitt TE, Caspi A, Belsky J, et al: Childhood experience and the onset of menarche: a test of a sociobiological model. Child Dev 63:47–58, 1992

Morrow AL, Devaud LL, Purdy RH, et al: Neuroactive steroid modulators of the stress response. Ann N Y Acad Sci 771:257–272, 1995

Morse CA, Dudley E, Guthrie J, et al: Relationships between premenstrual complaints and perimenopausal experiences. J Psychosom Obstet Gynaecol 19:182–191, 1998

Muse K: Hormonal manipulation in the treatment of premenstrual syndrome. Clin Obstet Gynecol 35:658–666, 1992

O'Boyle M, Severino SK, Hurt SW: Premenstrual syndrome and locus of control. Int J Psychiatry Med 18:67–74, 1988

Odber J, Cawood EHH, Bancroft J: Salivary cortisol in women with and without perimenstrual mood changes. J Psychosom Res 45:557–568, 1998

Palmer SA, Lambert MJ, Richards RL: The MMPI and premenstrual syndrome: profile fluctuations between best and worst times during the menstrual cycle. J Clin Psychol 47:215–221, 1991

Parry BL, Rosenthal NE, Tamarkin L, et al: Treatment of a patient with seasonal premenstrual syndrome. Am J Psychiatry 144:762–766, 1987

Parry BL, Hauger R, Lin E, et al: Neuroendocrine effects of light therapy in late luteal phase dysphoric disorder. Biol Psychiatry 36:356–364, 1994

Pearlstein TB, Stone AB, Lund SA, et al: Comparison of fluoxetine, bupropion, and placebo in the treatment of premenstrual dysphoric disorder. J Clin Psychopharmacol 17:261–266, 1997

Penland JG, Johnson PE: Dietary calcium and manganese effects on menstrual cycle symptoms. Am J Obstet Gynecol 168:1417–1423, 1993

Rabin DS, Schmidt PJ, Campbell G, et al: Hypothalamic-pituitary-adrenal function in patients with the premenstrual syndrome. J Clin Endocrinol Metab 71:1158–1162, 1990

Rapkin AJ, Morgan M, Goldman L, et al: Progesterone metabolite allopregnanolone in women with premenstrual syndrome. Obstet Gynecol 90:709–714, 1997

Reading AE: Cognitive model of premenstrual syndrome. Clin Obstet Gynecol 35:693–700, 1992

Richardson JTE: The premenstrual syndrome: a brief history. Soc Sci Med 41:761–767, 1995

Rickels K, Freeman E, Sondheimer S: Buspirone in treatment of premenstrual syndrome (letter). Lancet 1:777, 1989

Rivera-Tovar AD, Frank E: Late luteal phase dysphoric disorder in young women. Am J Psychiatry 147:1634–1636, 1990

Roca CA, Schmidt PJ, Rubinow DR: A follow-up study of premenstrual syndrome. J Clin Psychiatry 60:763–766, 1999

Rosenstein DL, Kalogeras KT, Kalafut M, et al: Peripheral measures of arginine vasopressin, atrial natriuretic peptide and adrenocorticotropic hormone in premenstrual syndrome. Psychoneuroendocrinology 21:347–359, 1996

Rothbaum BO, Jackson J: Religious influence on menstrual attitudes and symptoms. Women Health 16:63–78, 1990

Rubinow DR, Schmidt PJ: The neuroendocrinology of menstrual cycle mood disorders. Ann N Y Acad Sci 77:648–659, 1995

Sarno AP, Miller EJ, Lundblad EG: Premenstrual syndrome: beneficial effects of periodic low-dose danazol. Obstet Gynecol 70:33–36, 1987

Sayegh R, Schiff I, Wurtman J, et al: The effect of a carbohydrate-rich beverage on mood, appetite, and cognitive function in women with premenstrual syndrome. Obstet Gynecol 86:520–528, 1995

Schmidt PJ, Grover GN, Rubinow DR: Alprazolam in the treatment of premenstrual syndrome: a double-blind, placebo-controlled trial. Arch Gen Psychiatry 50:467–473, 1993

Schmidt PJ, Nieman LK, Danaceau MA, et al: Differential behavioral effects of gonadal steroids in women with and in those without premenstrual syndrome. N Engl J Med 338:209–216, 1998

Sothern RB, Slover GPT, Morris RW: Circannual and menstrual rhythm characteristics in manic eisodes and body temperature. Biol Psychiatry 33:194–203, 1993

Spitzer RL, Severino SK, Williams JBW, et al: Late luteal phase dysphoric disorder and DSM-III-R. Am J Psychiatry 146:892–897, 1989

Steege JF, Blumenthal JA: The effects of aerobic exercise on premenstrual symptoms in middle-aged women: a preliminary study. J Psychosom Res 37:127–133, 1993

Steiner M, Steinberg S, Stewart D, et al: Fluoxetine in the treatment of premenstrual dysphoria. N Engl J Med 332:1529–1534, 1995

Steiner M, Korzekwa M, Lamont J, et al: Intermittent fluoxetine dosing in the treatment of women with premenstrual dysphoria. Psychopharmacol Bull 33:771–774, 1997

Strassmann BI: The evolution of endometrial cycles and menstruation. Q Rev Biol 71:181–220, 1996

Sugawara M, Toda MA, Shima S, et al: Premenstrual mood changes and maternal mental health in pregnancy and the postpartum period. J Clin Psychol 53:225–232, 1997

Sundblad C, Modigh K, Andersch B, et al: Clomipramine effectively reduces premenstrual irritability and dysphoria: a placebo-controlled trial. Acta Psychiatr Scand 85:39–47, 1992

Sundblad C, Hedberg MA, Eriksson E: Clomipramine administered during the luteal phase reduces the symptoms of premenstrual syndrome: a placebo-controlled trial. Neuropsychopharmacology 9:133–145, 1993

Sundstrom I, Backstrom T: Citalopram increases pregnanolone sensitivity in patients with premenstrual syndrome: an open trial. Psychoneuroendocrinology 23:73–88, 1998

Sundstrom I, Ashbrook D, Backstrom T: Reduced benzodiazepine sensitivity in patients with premenstrual syndrome: a pilot study. Psychoneuroendocrinology 22:25–38, 1997

Sundstrom I, Andersson A, Nyberg S, et al: Patients with premenstrual syndrome have a different sensitivity to a neuroactive steroid during the menstrual cycle compared to control subjects. Neuroendocrinology 67:126–138, 1998

Sveinsdottir H: Prospective assessment of menstrual and premenstrual experiences of Icelandic women. Health Care Women Int 19:71–82, 1998

Thys-Jacobs S, Alvir J: Calcium regulating hormones across the menstrual cycle: evidence of a secondary hyperparathyroidism in women with PMS. J Clin Endocrinol Metab 80:2227–2232, 1995

Thys-Jacobs S, Starkey P, Bernstein D, et al: Calcium carbonate and the premenstrual syndrome: effects on premenstrual and menstrual symptoms. Am J Obstet Gynecol 179:444–452, 1998

Van den Akker OBA, Eves FF, Stein GS, et al: Genetic and environmental factors in premenstrual symptom reporting and its relationship to depression and a general neuroticism trait. J Psychosom Res 39:477–487, 1995

Wang M, Hammarback S, Lindhe BA, et al: Treatment of premenstrual syndrome by spironolactone: a double-blind, placebo-controlled study. Acta Obstet Gynecol Scand 74:803–808, 1995

Wang M, Seippel L, Purdy R, et al: Relationship between symptom severity and steroid variation in women with premenstrual syndrome: study on serum pregnenolone, pregnenolone sulfate, 5-alpha-pregnane-3,20-dione and 3-alpha-hydroxy-5-alpha-pregnan-20-one. J Clin Endocrinol Metab 81:1076–1082, 1996

Wurtman JJ: Carbohydrate craving: relationship between carbohydrate intake and disorders of mood. Drugs 39 (suppl 3):49–52, 1990

Yonkers KA: Anxiety symptoms and anxiety disorders: how are they related to premenstrual disorders? J Clin Psychiatry 58 (suppl 3):62–67, 1997a

Yonkers KA: The association between premenstrual dysphoric disorder and other mood disorders. J Clin Psychiatry 58 (suppl 15):19–25, 1997b

Yonkers KA, Halbreich U, Freeman E, et al: Symptomatic improvement of premenstrual dysphoric disorder with sertraline treatment. JAMA 278:983–988, 1997

Young SA, Hurt PH, Benedek DM, et al: Treatment of premenstrual dysphoric disorder with sertraline during the luteal phase: a randomized, double-blind, placebo-controlled crossover trial. J Clin Psychiatry 59:76–80, 1998

Index

*Page numbers printed in **boldface type refer to tables.***

Antipsychotic drugs, 14. *See also* individual drug names

Anxiety
  in cardiac allotransplantation, 9–10
  in organ pretransplant period, 82–83
  panic-level, 6
  as side effect of antihypertensive drugs, 12
  symptoms that present with cardiac symptoms, 10–11

Anxiety disorders, 10–11, 35, 50
  posttransplant, 95

Anxiolytics, for premenstrual syndrome, 120–121

Appetite, 81

Arrhythmias, 17

Aseptic meningitis, 88

Aspirin, 28

Asterixis, 43

Automatic internal cardioverter defibrillators (AICDs)
  behavior maintenance and, 5
  as life extender, 7
  postimplantation phase, 5–6
  psychiatric disorders in patients with, 5–7
  as source of security to patient, 6

Avoidant personality disorder, 118

Axis I and II disorders, in organ transplantation patient, 74–76

Azathioprine, 36, 86

Barrett's esophagus, 24

Bazett's formula, 13

Benzodiazepines, 51, 91
  for anxiety, 82

contraindications, 31–32, 45
  for hepatic encephalopathy, 45

Bethanechol, 24, 25

Bioterrism, xi

Bipolar illness, 50, 55
  menstruation and, 115

Brief Symptom Inventory, 56

Bulking agents, 41

Bupropion, 93
  in end-stage organ disease, **80**
  for premenstrual syndrome, 119
  for pretransplant depression, 79

Buspirone, 95, 121
  for anxiety, 82

CAD. *See* Coronary artery disease

Calcium, 14, 122

Cancer
  acute leukemia, 56
  of the colon, 36
  of the esophagus, 24
  gastric, 27–28
  hepatocellular, 48
  oropharyngeal, 56
  of the pancreas, 55–57

Carbamazepine, 16–17, 17, 29–30, 54

Carbohydrates, 122–123

Carcinoma. *See* Cancer

Cardiac allotransplantation
  long range, 10
  monitoring, 91
  opportunistic infections, 8
  postoperative period, 9
  prelisting psychiatric evaluation and waiting period, 8–9

Dicyclomine, 41
Diuretics, 17
Dopamine-2 receptors, 24
Doxepin, 30
Droperidol, 91
Drugs. *See also* individual drug
   names
   addictive anxiolytic, 6
   anticholinergic agents, 24
   antidepressant agents, 15–16
      in end-stage organ disease,
      80–81
   antiepileptic hypersensitivity
      syndrome, 54
   antipanic phamacotherapy, 41
   cardiovascular side effects of
      psychotropic medications,
      12–14, 12–17
   elimination, 51
   immunosuppressive agents,
      86–88
   injection drug use, 47
   interactions, 29–30, 79
   medications contributing to
      onset of delirium, **90**
   neuropsychiatric side effects of
      cardiovascular
      medications, 12
   nonsteroidal anti-
      inflammatory
      medications, 27
   opiates, 33
   for premenstrual syndrome,
      119–128
   promotility, 24–25, **25**
   psychotropic, hepatic diseases
      and, 50–52
Dual-phase spiral computed
   tomography scan, for
   diagnosis of carcinoma of the
   pancreas, 55–56

Dyspepsia, 30–34
Dysphagia, 24

ECG. *See* Electrocardiogram
EEG. *See* Electroencephalogram
Elderly patients
   delirium and, 89
   extrapyramidal symptoms,
      24–25
Electrocardiogram (ECG), 13
Electroencephalogram (EEG), 43
Electrolytes, 14
Employment status, 97–98
Encainide, 15–16
Endometriosis, 31
Endoscopic ultrasonography, for
   diagnosis of carcinoma of the
   pancreas, 55–56
Esomeprazole, 30
Esophagus
   cancer of, 24
   disorders, 23–27
   functional disorders, 26–27
   motility disorders, 24, 25–27
   nutcracker, 25–26
Essential circulatory
   hyperkinesis, 11
Estrogen, 116
Evening primrose oil, 127
Exercise, 124

Factitious disorder, 10
Family
   cardiac allotransplantation
      and, 10
   distress and, 8
Famotidine, side effects, 29
Fatigue, 12
FDA. *See* U.S. Food and Drug
   Administration
Fear, 9

Interferon alpha
  for hepatitis B and C, 48
  neuropsychiatric side effects,
    48–49
  side effects, **25**
Interpersonal therapy, 124
Intravenous hyperalimentation,
  37
Irritable bowel syndrome (IBS),
  27, 38–42
  classification, 38–39
  dietary management, 40–41
  Rome II criteria, **38**

Lactase-phlorizin hydrolase, 34
Lactose intolerance, 34
Lamotrigine, 54–55
Lansoprazole, 30
  for peptic ulcer disease, 29
Left ventricular assist devices
    (LVADs)
  psychiatric disorders in
    patients with, 7–8
  surgery and, 7
  "wearability," 7
Leptin, 113
Leuprolide acetate, 125
Lipid metabolism, alterations in,
  3
Lithium, 16, 17
Liver failure, 42, 44
  end-stage, 47–48
Locus of Control (test), 117
Loperamide, 41
Lorazepam, 29–30, 51, 82, 91
Luteal phase dosing, 119–120
LVADs. *See* Left ventricular assist
  devices

Macropsia, 11–12
Magnesium, 14

Magnetic resonance imaging, 87
  for functional bowel disorders,
    39
Malnutrition, 35
  stress and, ix
Manganese, 44
Maprotiline, 119
Marriage, cardiac
    allotransplantation and, 10
Medicare, 3
Medications. *See* Drugs;
    individual drug names
Medroxyprogesterone acetate,
  125–126
Men, couvade syndrome, 32
Menarche. *See* Menstruation
Menopause, 125
Menstruation, 113–128
  definition, 114
  menarche, 113
  nature of, 113
  premenstrual psychiatric
    disorders, 114–115
  premenstrual syndrome
    contributory factors, 116–
      118
    treatment, 119–128
  stress and, xi
Mental health professionals, 68,
  76
Mental retardation, 48
Mesalamine, 36
Metabolic encephalopathy, in
    postoperative cardiac
    allotransplantation, 9
Methadone, 74
Methylphenidate, 49, 94
Metoclopramide
  for delayed gastric emptying,
    34
  side effects, 24, **25**

Metronidazole, 36
for peptic ulcer disease, 29
MI. *See* Myocardial infarction
Micropsia, 11–12
Minnesota Multiphasic
Personality Inventory, 117
Mirtazapine, 93–94
for anxiety, 83
in end-stage organ disease, 81,
81
Modafinil, 94
Models
psychosomatic medicine, xiii–
xiv
stress-diathesis, 28
stress–vulnerability in illness,
ix
Mood disorders
stress and, x–xi
symptoms that present with
cardiac symptoms, 10–11
Mood stabilizers, 16–17
Moricizine, 15–16
Motor incoordination, 43
Mycophenolate mofetil, 86, 88
Myocardial infarction (MI), 3
Myo-inositol, 45

Narcotics, delirium and, **90**
Narcotics Anonymous, 73
National Health and Nutrition
Examination Survey III, 1
National Heart, Lung, and Blood
Institute, 7
Nefazodone, 53, 94, 119
in end-stage organ disease, **80**
for pretransplant depression,
79, 81
Neurocirculatory asthenia,
11
Neurocognitive recovery, 96

Neuroendocrinology,
premenstrual syndrome and,
116–117
Neuroleptics, 24, 91
cardiovascular side effects, 12–
14
for delirium, 90–91
Nizatidine, 29
NMDA. *See* N-methyl-D-
aspartate
N-methyl-D-aspartate (NMDA),
83
Nonsteroidal anti-inflammatory
medications, 27
Nortriptyline, 15, 16, 94
Nutcracker esophagus, 25–26
Nutrition
appetite, 81
dietary management in
irritable bowel syndrome,
40–41
food allergies, 34–35
in irritable bowel syndrome,
40–41
low-protein diet for hepatic
encephalopathy, 45
low-sodium diet, 17
premenstrual syndrome and,
121–122
renutrition for gastric
emptying, 34
ulcerative colitis and, 36–37

Octopamine, 44
OKT3, 88
Olanzapine, 14
Omega-6 essential fatty acids,
127
Omeprazole, 24, 30
for peptic ulcer disease, 29
Oophorectomy, 126

Opioids, 33
  dependence, 74
Oral contraceptives, 127–128
Organic mental syndromes, 8
Organ transplantation
  donor shortages, 68
  liver, 46–47, 52
  patient evaluation, 67–76
  perioperative period, 85–91
    intensive care unit
      environment, 85, **86**
  posttransplant period, 91–98
    neurocognitive recovery, 96
    psychological issues, 92–96
    quality of life, 96–98
  pretransplant waiting period,
    76–85
    anxiety, 82–83
    depression, 78–81, **80–81**
    medical issues and, 83–84
    psychological issues, 76–77
    social issues, 84–85
  psychiatric disorders in
    patients with, 3–10
  psychiatric overview, 67–98
  psychological issues, 92–96
  quality of life following, 75
  relapse, 72–73
  stress and, xi
  survival rates, 91–92
Orthostatic hypotension, 15
Osteoporosis, 122
Ostomy, 37–38
Oxazepam, 51
  for anxiety, 82
Oxidation, 51

Pacemakers, permanent
  adaptive phase
    (postimplantation), 4
  long-range phase, 4–5

perioperative phase, 4
  psychiatric disorders in
    patients with, 3–5
PACT. *See* Psychosocial
    Assessment of Candidates
    for Transplant
Pain
  abdominal, 30–34
  chronic, 92–93
  in intensive care unit, 85
  liver disease and, 48
  psychogenic, 10
  Rome II criteria for abdominal,
    31
Pain disorder, 11
Pancreas, carcinoma of, 55–57
Panic disorders, 26
  cancer and, 56
  gastrointestinal patients and,
    41, **41**
  pharmacotherapy, 41
Pantoprazole, 30
Paraneoplastic syndrome, 56
Parathyroid hormone, 57
Paroxetine, 16, 93, 119
  in end-stage organ disease, **80**
Patient, evaluation for organ
    transplantation, 67–76, **69–70**
  Axis I and II disorders, 74–76
  noncompliant, 71–72
  substance abuse and, 72–74
Pemoline, 53, 94
Peptic ulcer disease, 27–30
  medical treatment, 29–30
Peristalsis, 26
Personality disorders, 117–118
Phenothiazines, 14, 53
Phenylalanine, 44
Phenytoin, 54
Phototherapy, 124–125
Pimozide, 14

Warfarin, 17
White matter changes, 87
Women. *See also* Menstruation
  carcinoma of the pancreas and, 55
  constipation in, 33
  endometriosis, 31
  hysterectomy, 126
  menopause, 125
  oophorectomy, 126
  oral contraceptives and, 127–128
  osteoporosis and, 122
  pseudo–food allergy in, 34–35

Yeast β-galactosidase, 34

Zalephon, 29
Ziprasidone, 12–13, 14
Zolpidem, 29